OAPL

OXFORD AMERICAN PAIN LIBRARY

Perioperative Pain Management

Richard D. Urman, MD, MBA, CPE

Assistant Professor of Anesthesia
Director, Procedural Sedation Management and Safety
Brigham & Women's Hospital
Harvard Medical School
Boston, Massachusetts

Nalini Vadivelu, MD

Associate Professor of Anesthesiology
Department of Anesthesiology
Yale University School of Medicine
New Haven, Connecticut

Executive Series Editor

Russell K. Portenoy, MD

Chairman of the Department of Pain Medicine and Palliative Care
Beth Israel Medical Center
New York, NY

OXFORD
UNIVERSITY PRESS

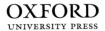

OXFORD
UNIVERSITY PRESS

Oxford University Press is a department of the University of Oxford.
It furthers the University's objective of excellence in research, scholarship,
and education by publishing worldwide.

Oxford   New York
Auckland   Cape Town   Dar es Salaam   Hong Kong   Karachi
Kuala Lumpur   Madrid   Melbourne   Mexico City   Nairobi
New Delhi   Shanghai   Taipei   Toronto

With offices in
Argentina   Austria   Brazil   Chile   Czech Republic   France   Greece
Guatemala   Hungary   Italy   Japan   Poland   Portugal   Singapore
South Korea   Switzerland   Thailand   Turkey   Ukraine   Vietnam

Oxford is a registered trademark of Oxford University Press in the UK
and certain other countries.

Published in the United States of America by
Oxford University Press
198 Madison Avenue, New York, NY 10016

Library of Congress Cataloging-in-Publication Data
Perioperative pain management / [edited by] Richard D. Urman, Nalini Vadivelu.
   p. ; cm.—(Oxford American pain library)
Includes bibliographical references and index.
ISBN 978-0-19-993721-9 (alk. paper)
I. Urman, Richard D.   II. Vadivelu, Nalini.   III. Series: Oxford American pain library.
[DNLM: 1. Pain Management—Handbooks.   2. Analgesics—therapeutic use—
Handbooks.   3. Anesthetics—therapeutic use—Handbooks.
4. Perioperative Care—Handbooks. WL 39]
LC Classification not assigned
616'.0472—dc23
2012046999

9 8 7 6 5 4 3 2 1
Printed in the United States of America
on acid-free paper

O A P L

OXFORD AMERICAN PAIN LIBRARY

Perioperative Pain Management

Dedication/Acknowledgment

I would like to dedicate this book to my colleagues among physicians, nurses, and physician assistants who over the years provided me with their invaluable advice and constant inspiration, to my wife Zina Matlyuk, MD for her support and patience while I was completing the manuscript, and to our daughter Abigail Rose.

Richard D. Urman, MD, MBA, CPE
Boston, Massachusetts

I dedicate this book to my teachers, colleagues and students, to my parents Major General Vadivelu and Gnanambigai, to my husband Thangamuthu Kodumudi and to my sons Gopal and Vijay for their constant encouragement.

Nalini Vadivelu, MD
New Haven, Connecticut

Table of Contents

Contributors

Vanita Ahuja, MD
Assistant Professor
Department of Anaesthesia
and Intensive Care
Government Medical College
and Hospital
Chandigarh, India

Wilson Almonte, MD
Resident, Department of
Anesthesiology
Albert Einstein College of Medicine -
Yeshiva University
Montefiore Medical Center
Bronx, New York

Orvil Ayala, MD
Resident, Department of
Anesthesiology
Albert Einstein College of Medicine -
Yeshiva University
Montefiore Medical Center
Bronx, New York

Veronica Carullo, MD
Director of Pediatric Pain Service
Assistant Professor, Department of
Anesthesiology
Assistant Professor, Department of
Pediatrics
Albert Einstein College of Medicine -
Yeshiva University
Montefiore Medical Center
Bronx, New York

Juan P. Cata, MD
Instructor
Department of Anesthesiology and
Perioperative Medicine
Division of Anesthesiology and
Critical Care
The University of Texas MD
Anderson Cancer Center
Houston, Texas

Sherif Costandi, MD
Pain Management Department
Cleveland Clinic
Cleveland, Ohio

Ehab Farag, MD, FRCA
Associate Professor
Staff Anesthesiologist
Department of Anesthesiology
Anesthesiology Institute
Cleveland Clinic
Cleveland, Ohio

Maged Guirguis, MD
Department of Pain Management
and Anesthesiology
Anesthesiology Institute
Cleveland Clinic
Cleveland, Ohio

Amitabh Gulati, MD
Assistant Professor
Department of Anesthesiology
and Critical Care
Memorial Sloan Kettering Cancer
Center
New York, New York

CONTRIBUTORS

Karina Gritsenko, MD
Assistant Professor, Department of
Anesthesiology
Albert Einstein College of
Medicine - Yeshiva University
Montefiore Medical Center
Bronx, New York

Boleslav Kosharskyy, MD
Assistant Professor, Department of
Anesthesiology
Albert Einstein College of
Medicine - Yeshiva University
Montefiore Medical Center
Bronx, New York

Zachary Leuschner, MD
Resident, Department of
Anesthesiology
Albert Einstein College of
Medicine - Yeshiva University
Montefiore Medical Center
Bronx, New York

**Christine Milner, MS, RN,
CPNP, CPON**
Nurse Practitioner, Pediatric Pain
Management Service
Department of Anesthesiology
Department of Pediatrics
Montefiore Medical Center
New York, New York

Sukanya Mitra, MD
Professor
Department of Anaesthesia and
Intensive Care
Government Medical College and
Hospital
Chandigarh, India

Nathaniel Pleasant, MD
Resident Physician
Department of Anesthesiology
Weill Medical College, Cornell
University
New York, New York

Richard W. Rosenquist, MD
Chairman
Department of Pain Management
Cleveland Clinic
Cleveland, Ohio

Atit Shah, MD
Resident, Department of
Anesthesiology
Albert Einstein College of
Medicine - Yeshiva University
Montefiore Medical Center
Bronx, New York

Naum Shaparin, MD
Director of Adult Pain Service
Assistant Professor, Department of
Anesthesiology
Assistant Professor, Department of
Family and Social Medicine
Albert Einstein College of
Medicine - Yeshiva University
Montefiore Medical Center
Bronx, New York

Dmitri Souzdalnitski, MD, PhD
Associate Staff
Department of Pain Management
Cleveland Clinic
Cleveland, Ohio

Yi Cai Isaac Tong, MD
Department of Anesthesiology,
Perioperative and Pain Medicine
Brigham and Women's Hospital
Harvard Medical School
Boston, Massachusetts

Travis Nickels, MD
Department of General
Anesthesiology
Anesthesiology Institute
Cleveland Clinic
Cleveland, Ohio

David B. Turk, MD
Resident, Department of
Anesthesiology
Albert Einstein College of
Medicine - Yeshiva University
Montefiore Medical Center
Bronx, New York

**Richard D. Urman, MD,
MBA, CPE**
Assistant Professor of Anesthesia
Director, Procedural Sedation
Management and Safety
Brigham & Women's Hospital
Harvard Medical School
Boston, Massachusetts

Nalini Vadivelu, MD
Associate Professor
Department of Anesthesiology
Yale University School of Medicine
New Haven, Connecticut

Amaresh Vydyanathan, MD, MS
Assistant Professor, Department of
Anesthesiology
Albert Einstein College of
Medicine - Yeshiva University
Montefiore Medical Center
Bronx, New York

Joseph Walker III, MD
Assistant Professor
Department of Orthopedics
University of Connecticut
Farmington, Connecticut

Roniel Weinberg, MD
Assistant Professor, Department of
Anesthesiology
Weill Medical College, Cornell
University
New York, New York

Alison Weisheipl, MD
Resident
Department of Anesthesiology,
Perioperative and Pain Medicine
Brigham and Women's Hospital
Boston, Massachusetts

Sherif Zaky, MD, PhD
Assistant Professor of Anesthesiology
Cleveland Clinic Lerner College of
Medicine of Case Western Reserve
University
Department of General
Anesthesiology
Anesthesiology Institute
Cleveland Clinic
Cleveland, Ohio

Chapter 1

Introduction to Acute Pain Management: A Team Approach

Boleslav Kosharskyy, Orvil Ayala, and Karina Gritsenko

Pain, as defined by the International Association for the Study of Pain (IASP), is an unpleasant sensory and emotional experience associated with actual or potential tissue damage. About one in four Americans have reported suffering from pain of any sort for more than 24 hours (1). In the perioperative setting, pain can be a manifestation of a preexisting pathology, the surgical procedure, or a combination of both. It is in this environment that the development of specialized teams dedicated to the treatment of pain is most needed. The objectives of this chapter are to discuss the origin of acute pain, to outline the organization of an acute pain service, and to describe different modalities available for the management of acute pain.

Pain in the Acute Setting

Acute pain is the normal, predicted physiologic response to a noxious chemical, thermal, or mechanical stimulus (2). For most patients the perception of postoperative pain is a major concern (3). Patients with postoperative pain account for approximately 60% of emergency department visits (4). Despite the efforts and innovations in pain management, many patients continue to experience intense pain after surgery (5).

The mechanism involved in the generation of pain originates from local inflammation and nerve damage typically associated with invasive procedures, trauma, and disease (2, 6). These processes result in the release of local mediators, including but are not limited to bradykinins, leukotrienes, 5-hydroxytryptamine, prostaglandins, substance P, and histamine (6). Nociceptors are sensory receptors that respond to these local mediators and send afferent (sensory) signals toward the spinal cord and then to the cerebral cortex (Fig. 1.1).

Due to the subjective component of pain perception, the assessment of pain and the treatment of pain rely heavily on the use of self-report pain scales. These scales have been well validated in both the research and clinical settings (7). One-dimensional self-report pain scales may be used in patients with an obvious source of pain (6). Examples of one-dimensional self-report pain scales include verbal rating scales (VRS), numeric rating scales (NRS), and visual analog scales (VAS; Fig. 1.2).

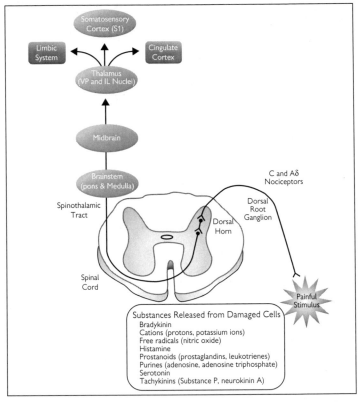

Figure 1.1 Diagram of Ascending Pain Pathway (Sigma Aldrich). Available at: http://www.sigmaaldrich.com/life-science/cell-biology/learning-center/pathway-slides-and/ascending-pain-pathway.html.

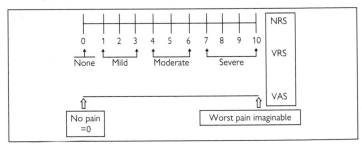

Figure 1.2 Example of One-dimensional Self-Reporting Pain Scales. Available at: http://www.medscape.com/viewarticle/580952_2.

Multidimensional self-report pain scales, such as the McGill Pain Questionnaire and the Brief Pain Inventory (Fig. 1.3), are better when used for the assessment of patients with complex pain (6).

The inadequate relief of pain may result in significant complications; some of the key examples are listed in Table 1.1.

Form 3.2 **Brief pain inventory**

Date ___ /___ /___ Time:_____

Name: _____
　　　　　Last　　　　　First　　　Middle Initial

1) Throughout our lives, most of us have had pain from time to time (such as minor headaches, sprains, and toothaches). Have you had pain other than these everyday kinds of pain today?

　　　　1. Yes　　　2. No

2) On the diagram, shade in the areas where you feel pain. Put an X on the area that hurts the most.

3) Please rate your pain by circling the one number that best describes your pain at its **worst** in the last 24 hours.

0　1　2　3　4　5　6　7　8　9　10
No Pain　　　　　　　　　　　Pain as bad as you can imagine

4) Please rate your pain by circling the one number that best describes your pain at its **least** in the last 24 hours.

0　1　2　3　4　5　6　7　8　9　10
No Pain　　　　　　　　　　　Pain as bad as you can imagine

5) Please rate your pain by circling the one number that best describes your pain on the **average.**

0　1　2　3　4　5　6　7　8　9　10
No Pain　　　　　　　　　　　Pain as bad as you can imagine

6) Please rate your pain by circling the one number that tells how much pain you have **right now.**

0　1　2　3　4　5　6　7　8　9　10
No Pain　　　　　　　　　　　Pain as bad as you can imagine

7) What treatments or medications are you receiving for your pain?

_____

_____

8) In the last 24 hours, how much relief have pain treatments or medications provided? Please circle the one percentage that shows how much **relief** you have received.

0% 10　20　30　40　50　60　70　80　90　100%
No Relief　　　　　　　　　　　Complete Relief

9) Circle the one number that describes how, during the past 24 hours, pain has interfered with your:

A. General activity

0　1　2　3　4　5　6　7　8　9　10
Does not interfere　　　　　　　Completely interferes

B. Mood

0　1　2　3　4　5　6　7　8　9　10
Does not interfere　　　　　　　Completely interferes

C. Walking ability

0　1　2　3　4　5　6　7　8　9　10
Does not interfere　　　　　　　Completely interferes

D. Normal work (includes both work outside the home and housework)

0　1　2　3　4　5　6　7　8　9　10
Does not interfere　　　　　　　Completely interferes

E. Relations with other people

0　1　2　3　4　5　6　7　8　9　10
Does not interfere　　　　　　　Completely interferes

F. Sleep

0　1　2　3　4　5　6　7　8　9　10
Does not interfere　　　　　　　Completely interferes

G. Enjoyment of life

0　1　2　3　4　5　6　7　8　9　10
Does not interfere　　　　　　　Completely interferes

Figure 1.3 Brief Pain Inventory. Available at: http://www.medscape.com/viewarticle/585568.

Table 1.1　Some Complications of Inadequate Pain Relief	
Increased stay in post-anesthesia care unit	Development of chronic pain
Delayed discharge to home	Decreased patient satisfaction
Unanticipated hospital readmission	Delayed return to normal activities of daily living
Increased cost of care	Decreased quality of life
Modified from Joshi et al. ACNA 2005;23:21–36.	

Table 1.2 Potential Barriers to the Effective Treatment of Pain

Inadequate patient education regarding pain and its management	Deficits in pain management education of healthcare providers
Providers' and administrators' ignorance of proper pain management protocols and responsibilities	Lack of an interdisciplinary plan and exchange of ideas for the proper management in pain

Modified from the IASP's Global Year Against Acute Pain 2010–2011, *Interventions: Benefits and Barriers*, 2010. Available at: http://www.iasp-pain.org/AM/Template.cfm?Section=Fact_Sheets3&Template=/CM/ContentDisplay.cfm&ContentID=11784. Accessibility verified February 6, 2013.

Painful conditions have led to the loss of productive hours, with estimated costs of about $61.2 billion per year (8). In 2008, annual spending by federal and state governments for the treatment of pain was estimated at $99 billion, and the burden on society was estimated to be about $560 to 635 billion (9).

There are many barriers to providing adequate pain management (Table 1.2).

Lack of specialized task forces for pain treatment has led to patient dissatisfaction as well as lower patient expectations with regard to pain relief (10). In 2001, the Joint Commission on Accreditation of Healthcare Organizations established standards for the management of pain. These standards require organizations to recognize the patient's right to the assessment and management of pain; screen patients at regular intervals and reassess periodically for pain; and educate patients and their families about pain management (11). In 2004, the American Society of Anesthesiologists Task Force revised its practice guidelines for acute pain management. These guidelines encouraged the development of multidisciplinary teams dedicated to the treatment of pain as well as the education of other house staff on the assessment and management of pain in the acute setting.

Acute Pain Service Teams

The creation of an acute pain service (APS) dedicated to the management of acute pain was proposed over 50 years ago (12), but the first documented experiences with an APS were published in 1988 (13). According to the Royal College of Anaesthetists, the items listed in Table 1.3 are needed to provide effective and safe management of acute pain (14).

Table 1.3 Requirements for the Safe and Effective Management of Acute Pain

Acute Pain Management Service	Ongoing education and training for all healthcare staff involved in the management of acute pain patients
Multidisciplinary team (medical, nursing, pharmacy)	A named physician to direct the APS
Input from other healthcare professionals (e.g., physical therapy)	APS availability at all times
Written guidelines and protocols for the acute management of patients	Adequate accommodation and facilities for the care of acute pain

Modified from the Royal College of Anaesthetists, Acute pain services, 2010.

The roles played by each member of the APS are of great importance, and key points are highlighted in Table 1.4.

The APS allows for an environment in which acute pain may be managed efficiently to decrease the complications and discomfort patients experience while in pain. The improvements in patient care with an APS may lead to an increase in the quality of life for the patient, an increase in patient satisfaction, and a decrease in readmissions secondary to unrelieved pain (14). A study involving 1,518 surgical inpatients showed that perception of pain had significantly improved since the implementation of an APS (15). Some of the benefits of an effective APS are listed in Table 1.5.

Services Provided by the APS

A multitude of techniques may be offered to a patient in acute pain, ranging from noninvasive techniques, such as patient education and administration of oral medications, to invasive techniques, such as intravenous administration of

Table 1.4 Roles of the APS Members

Director of the APS

- Sets and coordinates the direction and goals for the APS
- Creates and implements the protocols and policies for the APS
- Reviews the cases for quality assurance/quality improvement

APS Attending Physicians

- In charge of patient rounds and supervise procedures and consultations

Residents' and Fellows' Involvement in the APS

- In charge of rounding on patients daily, responding to consults, performing procedures, and being available for patients when on call

Nurses' Involvement In the APS

- Advanced practice nurse: in charge of coordinating continuity of care, designing in-services for nurses and patients, assisting in development of the goals, policies, and protocols
- Acute pain nurse: in charge of assessing the effects of analgesia and adjusting pain therapy according to protocols

Modified from Viscusi et al. *Organization of an acute pain management service incorporating regional anesthesia techniques.* NYSORA, 2009. Available at: http://www.nysora.com/pain_pain_management/3055-organization_acute_acute_pain_management.html.

Table 1.5 Some Institutional Benefits of Having an Effective APS

Decreased hospital stay or ICU stay
Decreased use of hospital resources
Improved hospital reputation and marketability
Fewer patient complications (e.g., acute pain → chronic pain)
Fewer days of disability and loss of productivity for patients
Decreased cost to insurance companies

Modified from the IASP's Global Year Against Acute Pain 2010–2011, *Interventions: Benefits and Barriers,* 2010. Available at: http://www.iasp-pain.org/AM/Template.cfm?Section=Fact_Sheets3& Template=/CM/ContentDisplay.cfm&ContentID=11784. Accessibility verified February 6, 2013.

medications, nerve blocks, patient-controlled analgesia (PCA), and neuraxial procedures. Some of the interventions undertaken by the APS are highlighted in Table 1.6.

Patient education and realistic expectations about postoperative pain have been shown to allow the patient to cope with pain and other postoperative discomforts as compared to uninformed patients (16, 17). Patients should be taught how to express their pain by using the self-report pain scales discussed above as well as how to use a PCA pump if they are likely to receive one (17). In general, the goal of a PCA is to allow the patient to independently administer analgesics based on his or her current state of pain. This method of acute pain management avoids the extreme swings in plasma levels of analgesics that may lead to adverse effects (e.g., respiratory depression) that are more likely to occur with the systemic dosing of analgesics (18). Guidelines for PCA delivery of medications are highlighted in Table 1.7.

Systemic analgesic options, whether administered orally, intravenously, or intramuscularly, may include opioids, nonsteroidal anti-inflammatories (NSAIDs), or adjuncts such as ketamine, α2-agonists, or local anesthetics. Opioids have long been the mainstay of therapy for the treatment of acute postoperative pain, especially for patients who are experiencing moderate to severe pain (19). Multimodal analgesic techniques have aimed at minimizing the use of opioids as sole therapy, thus allowing for the use of other analgesics such as NSAIDs as either sole therapy or as adjuncts to opioids (20). NSAIDs generally act by inhibiting prostaglandins in the periphery (the area where trauma has

Table 1.6 Possible APS Interventions for the Management of Acute Pain

Educating the patient	Continuous epidural analgesia
Nerve blocks or medications prior to incision	Single-shot neuraxial opioids
Opioids and intravenous patient-controlled analgesia	Patient-controlled epidural analgesia
Nonsteroidal anti-inflammatory drugs	Continuous peripheral nerve analgesia (catheters)

Modified from the IASP's Global Year Against Acute Pain 2010–2011, *Interventions: Benefits and Barriers*, 2010. Available at: http://www.iasp-pain.org/AM/Template.cfm?Section=Fact_Sheets3&Template=/CM/ContentDisplay.cfm&ContentID=11784. Accessibility verified February 6, 2013.

Table 1.7 Guidelines for Medications Used for an IV PCA

Drug Concentration	Bolus Size	Lockout Interval (in minutes)	Continuous Infusion
Morphine (1 mg/mL)	0.5–2.5 mg	6–10	1–2 mg/hr
Fentanyl (0.01 mg/mL)	20–50 mcg	5–10	10–100 mcg/hr
Hydromorphone (0.2 mg/mL)	0.05–0.25 mg	10–20	0.2–0.4 mg/hr
Methadone (1 mg/mL)	0.5–1.5 mg	10–30	–
Sufentanil (0.002 mg/mL)	2–5 mcg	4–10	2–8 mcg/hr

Modified from Hurley R, Meredith A Chapter 40: Perioperative Pain Management. In Miller R, Pardo M, eds. *Basics of Anesthesia*, 6th ed. Philadelphia: Saunders, 2011: 650–662.

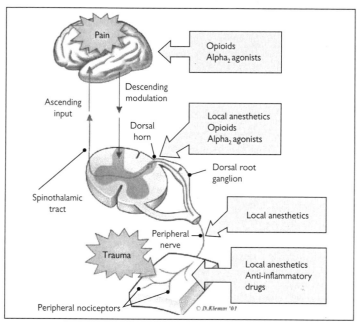

Figure 1.4 Illustration of Site of Action of Medications Used for the Treatment of Acute Pain. Available at: http://www.cybermedicine2000.com/pharmacology2000/Central/Opioids/opioidiv2.htm.

occurred) and have been shown to work well in patients experiencing mild to moderate pain. Figure 1.4 illustrates the site of action of some of the medications used in the treatment of acute postoperative pain.

Several neuraxial techniques may be used for the treatment of acute pain. Such examples include single-shot neuraxial opioids, continuous epidural analgesia, and patient-controlled epidural analgesia. Some of the indications for these techniques include surgeries involving the thoracic region, abdominal region, and/or lower extremities. Contraindications include patient refusal, coagulopathy, bacteremia, and localized infections at the area of needle insertion (21). These techniques are of great benefit to the patient as they provide greater analgesia, improve pulmonary function, are associated with fewer cardiac complications, and allow for a quicker recovery (22). The APS should always directly supervise the management of epidural analgesics in the postoperative state to ensure adequate pain relief and proper functioning of the catheter and pump and to address any complex adverse reaction that may occur secondary to this invasive technique and medications involved (23). Guidelines for the neuraxial analgesics are highlighted in Table 1.8.

Peripheral nerve-blocking techniques in the treatment of acute postoperative pain are especially advantageous if there are contraindications to neuraxial techniques (24). They provide great pain control in the immediate postoperative state, and if combined with an insertion of peripheral nerve catheter they may provide great analgesia for a more prolonged period (25). Patients must remain hospitalized while the continued peripheral nerve analgesic technique is stabilized; one of the ways of ensuring effective therapy is highlighted in Table 1.9 (25).

Infusion pumps can be used at home and allow the patient to take advantage of the continued analgesic therapy once discharged from the hospital as well as when undergoing physical therapy (25).

Conclusion

The unified concern for the treatment of acute pain in the perioperative setting has helped create an allegiance of responsible healthcare providers who work together for the sole purpose of decreasing the complications and discomfort experienced by postoperative patients. The multifaceted approach provided by an APS allows for the best treatment of patients with acute postoperative pain. With the continued efforts of the APS in helping to educate, train, and collaborate with both patients and other healthcare workers, the goals of increasing the quality of life and patient satisfaction appear promising.

Table 1.8 Guidelines for Neuraxial Analgesics Used

Drug	Single-Shot Spinal Dose	Single-Shot Epidural Dose	Epidural Infusion Rate
Opioids or Derivatives of Opioids			
Fentanyl	5–25 mcg	50–100 mcg	25–100 mcg/hr
Sufentanil	2–10 mcg	10–50 mcg	10–20 mcg/hr
Morphine	0.1–0.3 mg	1–5 mg	0.1–1 mg/hr
Hydromorphone	–	0.5–1 mg	0.1–0.2 mg/hr
Meperidine	–	20–60 mg	10–60 mg/hr
Local Anesthetics			
Bupivacaine	5–15 mg	25–150 mg	1–25 mg/hr
Ropivacaine	–	25–200 mg	6–20 mg/hr
Adjuncts			
Clonidine	–	100–900 mcg	10–50 mcg/hr

Modified from Hurley R, Meredith A. Chapter 40: Perioperative Pain Management. In Miller R, Pardo M, eds. *Basics of Anesthesia*, 6th ed. Philadelphia: Saunders, 2011:650–662.

Table 1.9 One Method of Stabilizing the Treatment of Acute Postoperative Pain with the use of Continuous Peripheral Nerve Catheter Infusion

Initial Therapy:
Bupivacaine 0.1% at 10–20 mL/hr
If Initial Therapy is Not Effective:
Try a higher concentration of bupivacaine, such as 0.25%
And/or administer a bolus injection of 20 mL of 0.25% to 0.35%

Modified from Ballantyne J, Ryder E. Chapter 21: Acute Pain. In Ballantyne J, ed. *The Massachusetts General Hospital Handbook of Pain Management*, 3rd ed. Philadelphia: Lippincott Williams & Wilkins, 2006:299.

References

1. National Center for Health Statistics. *Health, Unites States, 2006. With Chart book on Trends in the Health of Americans.* Hyattsville, MD, 2006.

2. Mahajan G, Holtsman M. Major opioids in pain management. In: Benzon H, Fishman S, Raja S, Cohen S, Liu S, eds. *Essentials of Pain Medicine.* 3rd Ed. Philadelphia, PA: Saunders, 2011, 86.

3. Joshi G, Ogunnaike B. Consequences of inadequate postoperative pain relief and chronic persistent postoperative pain. *Anesthesiology Clinics of North America.* 2005;23(1):21–36.

4. Cordell W, Keene K, Giles B, Jones JB, Jones JH, Brizendine E. The high prevalence of pain in emergency medical care. *American Journal of Emergency Medicine* 2002;20(3):165–169.

5. Apfelbaum J, Chen, Mehta S, Gan T. Postoperative Pain Experience: Results from a National Survey Suggest Postoperative Pain Continues to Be Undermanaged. *Anesthesia & Analgesia* 2003;97(2):534–540.

6. Gandhi K, Heitz JW, Viscusi ER. Challenges in acute pain management. *Anesthesiology Clinics* 2011;29(2):291–309.

7. Edward RR, Berde C. Pain assessment. In: Benzon H, Fishman S, Raja S, Cohen S, Liu S, eds. *Essentials of Pain Medicine.* 3rd Ed. Philadelphia, PA: Saunders, 2011, 28.

8. Stewart WF, Ricci JA, Chee E, Morganstein D. Lost productive work time costs from health conditions in the United States: Results from the American Productivity Audit. *Journal of Occupational and Environmental Medicine* 2003;45(12):1234–1246.

9. Institute of Medicine of the National Academies. *Relieving Pain in America: A Blueprint for Transforming Prevention, Care, Education, and Research.* Washington, DC: The National Academies Press, 2011.

10. Carr, E. Barriers to effective pain management. *Journal of Perioperative Practice* 2007;17(5):200–203, 206–208.

11. JCAHO. Facts about pain management, 2012. Available at: http://www.jointcommission.org/pain_management. Accessibility verified January 2, 2013.

12. Avery-Jones F. Postoperative pain. In: Bailey H, ed. *Pye's Surgical Handicraft.* Bristol, UK: Wright, 1961, 197–206.

13. Ready LB, Oden R, Chadwick HS, Benedetti C, Rooke GA, Caplan R, Wild LM. Development of an anesthesiology-based postoperative pain management service. *Anesthesiology* 1988;68(1):100–106.

14. Acute Pain Services, revised 2010: Guidance on the provision of anesthesia services for acute pain management. The Royal College of Anesthetists. Available at: www.rcoa.ac.uk/system/files/CSQ-GPAS6-AcutePain.pdf. Accessibility verified January 2, 2013.

15. Tighe SQ, Bie JA, Nelson RA, Skues MA. The acute pain service: effective or expensive care? *Anaesthesia* 1998;53(4):397–403.

16. Egbert LD, Battit GE, Welch CE, Bartlett MK. Reduction of postoperative pain by encouragement and instruction of patients: A study of doctor–patient rapport. *New England Journal of Medicine* 1964;270:825–827.

17. Ballantyne JC. Management of acute postoperative pain. In: Longnecker DE, Brown DL, Newman MF, Zapol WM, eds. *Anesthesiology* 1st Ed. New York, NY: The McGraw-Hill Companies, 2008, 1717.

18. Ballantyne JC, Ryder E. Postoperative pain in adults. In: Ballantyne JC, ed. *The Massachusetts General Hospital Handbook of Pain Management.* 3rd Ed. Philadelphia, PA: Lippincott, Williams and Wilkins, 2006, 288.

19. Ballantyne JC, Ryder E. Postoperative pain in adults. In: Ballantyne JC, ed. *The Massachusetts General Hospital Handbook of Pain Management.* 3rd Ed. Philadelphia, PA: Lippincott, Williams and Wilkins, 2006, 284.

20. Ballantyne JC, Ryder E. Postoperative pain in adults. In: Ballantyne JC, ed. *The Massachusetts General Hospital Handbook of Pain Management.* 3rd Ed. Philadelphia, PA: Lippincott, Williams and Wilkins, 2006, 283–284.

21. Ballantyne JC. Management of acute postoperative pain. In: Longnecker DE, Brown DL, Newman MF, Zapol WM, eds. *Anesthesiology* 1st Ed. New York, NY: The McGraw-Hill Companies, 2008, 1726.

22. Ballantyne JC, Ryder E. Postoperative pain in adults. In: Ballantyne JC, ed. *The Massachusetts General Hospital Handbook of Pain Management* 3rd Ed. Philadelphia, PA: Lippincott, Williams and Wilkins, 2006, 290.

23. Ballantyne JC, Ryder E. Postoperative pain in adults. In: Ballantyne JC, ed. *The Massachusetts General Hospital Handbook of Pain Management* 3rd Ed. Philadelphia, PA: Lippincott, Williams and Wilkins, 2006, 291.

24. Ballantyne JC. Management of acute postoperative pain. In: Longnecker DE, Brown DL, Newman MF, Zapol WM, eds. *Anesthesiology* 1st Ed. New York, NY: The McGraw-Hill Companies, 2008, 1730.

25. Ballantyne JC, Ryder E. Postoperative pain in adults. In: Ballantyne JC, ed. *The Massachusetts General Hospital Handbook of Pain Management* 3rd Ed. Philadelphia, PA: Lippincott, Williams and Wilkins, 2006, 299.

Chapter 2

Mechanisms of Pain

Sukanya Mitra, Vanita Ahuja, Richard D. Urman, and Nalini Vadivelu

Pain: Definition, Functions, and Types

According to the International Association for the Study of Pain (IASP), pain is "an unpleasant sensory and emotional experience associated with actual or potential tissue damage, or described in terms of such damage." Pain, especially acute nociceptive pain, has certain adaptive functions, such as identifying and localizing noxious stimuli; initiating withdrawal responses that limit tissue injury and protect the patient from further damage; inhibiting mobility, thereby enhancing wound healing and controlling inflammation; and initiating motivational and affective responses that modify future behavior.

On the other hand, there can be maladaptive consequences of prolonged severe untreated pain. It can increase postoperative or traumatic morbidity; delay recovery, with further untoward consequences (physical, emotional, financial, and social); lead to development of chronic pain; and cause physiologically unnecessary suffering.

Perioperative pain is one of most common types of acute nociceptive-inflammatory pain, which, if not properly controlled, can lead to any or all of these maladaptive consequences. Thus, it is important to appreciate the basic mechanisms of pain and how to target perioperative pain. Each of the four types of pain is outlined below (1).

Nociceptive pain is physiologic pain produced by noxious stimuli that activate high-threshold nociceptor neurons. It is transient, proportionate to the noxious stimulus, there is no hypersensitivity of the pain system, no lesions or dysfunction of the central nervous system (CNS), and the pain serves an adaptive function (protection of the organism from the noxious stimulus).

Inflammatory pain is pain hypersensitivity due to peripheral tissue inflammation involving the detection of active inflammation by nociceptors and a sensitization of the nociceptive system. The purpose is to promote healing of injured tissue. As in nociceptive pain, there are no lesions or dysfunction of the CNS and the pain serves an adaptive function (promotion of healing). The difference from nociceptive pain is that in inflammatory pain, there is hypersensitivity of the pain system due to increased excitability of the primary peripheral nerve terminals to stimuli that ordinarily are not noxious (i.e., peripheral sensitization; see later).

Neuropathic pain, according to the IASP definition, is "pain initiated or caused by a pathologic lesion or dysfunction" in the peripheral nerves and CNS. Common examples are diabetic neuropathic pain, postherpetic pain, trigeminal neuralgia, and pain related to stroke, multiple sclerosis, or spinal cord injury. Neuropathic pain is maladaptive because it does not serve the purpose of either protection from noxious stimuli or promotion of healing.

Functional (or dysfunctional) pain is also maladaptive and hence pathological pain, defined as "amplification of nociceptive signaling in the absence of either inflammation or neural lesions" (1). Unlike neuropathic pain, here there is no known peripheral or CNS lesion or damage. Examples include fibromyalgia, irritable bowel syndrome, and interstitial cystitis.

Pain: Anatomy and Physiology

The anatomy of pain is composed of an ascending pathway (main function: relaying the pain-related nerve impulse from the periphery to the brain) and the descending pathway (main function: supraspinal modulation of pain processing and perception) (2). Brain areas concerned with pain serve the main functions of pain perception, modulation, affective, and behavioral components of pain. Besides these, other components of the pain anatomy (main function: pain modulation) include spinal interneurons, the glial system, and the sympathetic nervous system.

The **ascending pathway** is a three-neuron pathway starting from the periphery, traveling through the peripheral nerve and the dorsal horn of the spinal cord, ascending through the spinal cord, and reaching the thalamus and finally the cerebral cortex.

The first-order neuron (also called primary/peripheral sensory neuron or nociceptor neuron or simply nociceptor) starts at the periphery from the peripheral nerve terminals. The cell body is in the dorsal root ganglion just outside the dorsal part of the spinal cord. It enters the spinal cord through the dorsal root and synapses through its central nerve terminals with the second-order neuron at the superficial lamina of the dorsal horn of the spinal cord.

The second-order neuron (also called secondary neuron, projection neuron, transmission neuron, dorsal horn neuron, or spinal neuron) starts in the dorsal horn of the spinal cord, crosses over to the contralateral side, ascends up the spinal cord, and typically terminates in the thalamus or other brain areas such as the parabrachial area (PBA).

The third-order neuron (also called tertiary neuron) starts from the thalamus and terminates in the cerebral cortex (responsible for the sensory localization and discriminatory aspects of the pain perception); or starts from the PBA and ends in the limbic system (responsible for the affective aspects of pain).

The descending pathways are composed of two functional types: facilitatory (enhances pain perception) and inhibitory (decreases pain perception). They start from brain areas such as limbic system, PBA, peri-aqueductal gray, nucleus raphe magnus, and finally the rostral ventromedial medulla. They converge on the synapses (both presynaptic and postsynaptic) between the first- and second-order neurons in the dorsal horn of the spinal cord. They modulate the upward transmission of the pain impulses in a facilitatory or inhibitory manner.

There is no single "pain center" in the brain; rather, there are interconnected areas in the cerebral cortex where different aspects of pain are perceived (the "pain matrix"). The pain matrix is composed of cerebral cortical areas where the third-order neurons terminate: primary and secondary somatosensory cortex, insular cortex, anterior cingulate cortex, and prefrontal cortex. The primary and secondary somatosensory cortex is concerned with the sensory, perceptual, localizing, and discriminatory aspects of pain experience. In contrast, areas such as the insular cortex, anterior cingulate cortex, limbic system, and hypothalamus are concerned with the affective, emotional, and behavioral aspects of pain. Other brain areas are concerned with the origin of the descending pathway of pain, as mentioned above.

In addition to the above, there are some other areas or components of pain anatomy. These are the spinal interneurons (excitatory or inhibitory), which connect some of the first-order and second-order neurons in the dorsal horn of the spinal cord; glial cells, such as astrocytes and microglia (along with interneurons, these play an important role in central pain sensitization and neuropathic pain); and the sympathetic nervous system (in acute inflammatory pain, it releases the neurotransmitters epinephrine and norepinephrine in the locally inflamed area and thus contributes to the "inflammatory soup"; it can also be involved in several chronic pain syndromes).

Stages of the Nociceptive Process

The stages of the nociceptive process are as follows:

- Transduction: The process by which noxious stimuli (mechanical, thermal, chemical) acting on the peripheral nociceptor terminals are converted ("transduced") into electrical activity within the terminals, finally culminating in an action potential nerve impulse
- Conduction: The process by which the nerve pulse travels (is "conducted") through the length of the first-order neuron to reach the synapse with the second-order neuron
- Transmission: The process by which synaptic transfer of information takes place at the synapse between the first- and second-order neurons in the dorsal horn of the spinal cord
- Perception: The actual conscious experience of the pain, both its sensory (localization, character, discrimination) and its affective (emotional) aspects
- Modulation: Pain experience is not a passive and proportionate mechanical response to the noxious stimuli. A multitude of factors actively moderate ("modulate") the stimulus-response pathway. As a broad umbrella term, pain modulation denotes the processes that affect and change the above four steps.

Transduction

In transduction, primary noxious stimuli act on receptors/ion channels on peripheral nociceptor terminals, causing intracellular cation (Ca^{++} and Na^+)

entry, leading to membrane depolarization ("generator potentials"). Summation of these small generator potentials further leads to activation of voltage-gated sodium channels until there is generation of action potential (nerve impulse). These self-propagating nerve impulses reach the other end (central terminal) of the peripheral nociceptor neuron. The primary noxious stimuli can be severe heat (>42 degrees C) or cold (<10 degrees C), traumatic or potentially tissue-injuring mechanical force, or irritant chemicals. The receptors/ion channels specifically expressed on the peripheral nociceptor terminals for pain signal detection are composed mostly of the family of transient receptor potential vanilloid (TRPV) calcium ion channels, and also the P2 family of purinoceptors for adenosine triphosphate (ATP), acid-sensitive ion channels, and so forth. These are high-threshold ion channels, activated only by stimuli that actually cause, or have the potential to cause, tissue injury.

Under ordinary conditions, low-intensity or non-noxious stimuli do not transduce these ion channels/receptors. During ongoing trauma or inflammation, however, further changes take place in the periphery, which reduce the threshold of these transducers. Then ordinarily non-noxious stimuli can also be transduced into nerve impulses ("peripheral sensitization").

Conduction

Conduction is the passage of electrical activity (action potentials) from the peripheral to the central terminal of the primary afferent sensory neuron. There are three types of primary afferent nerve fibers: Aβ, Aδ, and C (Table 2.1). Aδ and C fibers carry pain sensation from the periphery to the center (i.e., these are the first-order neurons/nociceptors). Aβ fibers typically do not carry pain sensation. In neuropathic pain, however, sensation carried by them can also be interpreted as pain sensation or otherwise unpleasant sensation (dysesthesia). Aδ fibers, being thinly myelinated, transmit pain faster than the unmyelinated C fibers, resulting in a rapid-onset (<1 s), well-localized, sharp or stinging sensation of short duration ("first pain"). Its functions are to immediately alert the organism to actual or potential injury; to localize the site of injury; and to initiate reflex withdrawal responses to protect the organism. C fibers are unmyelinated and have a high threshold, are usually polymodal (i.e., respond nonspecifically to thermal, mechanical, or chemical modalities of stimuli, provided these are strong enough), and cause a delayed (seconds to minutes) perception of pain described as a diffuse burning, stabbing sensation that is often prolonged and may become progressively more uncomfortable ("second pain").

Table 2.1 Types of Primary Sensory Afferent Fibers			
	Aβ	**Aδ**	**C**
Myelination	Yes	Yes (thinly)	No
Diameter (μ)	6–12	2–5	0.2–1.5
Conduction speed (m/s)	30–50	5–25	<2
Threshold for stimulation	Low	High	High
Activated by	Touch, vibration	Noxious stimuli	Noxious stimuli

Transmission

The synapse between the first-order and second-order neurons (either directly or via a short interneuron) in the dorsal horn of the spinal cord is vital for transmission of pain impulses further and alteration of the pain signal characteristics (spinal pain modulation, "central sensitization" [see below]). First-order neurons predominantly release the excitatory neurotransmitter glutamate in the synaptic cleft. Second-order neurons have glutamatergic and many other receptors, which receive their respective ligands from other sources such as excitatory and inhibitory spinal interneurons, glial cells (astrocytes and microglia), other local neurons, and descending pathway neurons from higher brain centers (peri-aqueductal gray, rostral ventromedial medulla). The second-order projection neurons integrate inputs from all these sources, and the final resultant electrical activity is transmitted upward through the ascending pathway to the thalamus and other centers (e.g., PBA) in the brain.

Ascending Pathway in the Spinal Cord

Some second-order neurons make connection with sympathetic anterolateral horn cells, resulting in sympathetic autonomic response, and motor anterior horn cells, responsible for reflex withdrawal and hypertonia. Other second-order neurons cross over and continue upward through the contralateral ascending spinal tracts. The most important tract is lateral spinothalamic tract, which terminates in the thalamus. This is important for the perception of pain. Other ascending tracts, such as spinoreticular and spinomesencephalic tracts, terminate in the thalamus but also make connections with centers in the midbrain (PBA, peri-aqueductal gray, nucleus raphe magnus). These are important for the affective aspect of pain.

Mechanisms of Pain

These may be conceptualized as follows: (a) events occurring at the peripheral terminal of nociceptors during acute pain, (b) peripheral sensitization, and (c) central sensitization. These are the main mechanisms underlying nociceptive-inflammatory pain, of which perioperative pain is the prototype (3–5). Other important mechanisms of pain do exist (e.g., phenotypic switch, spinal interneuronal disinhibition, structural reorganization, neural-glial-immune interaction, etc.), but those are of greater importance in chronic or neuropathic pain and hence will not be pursued here further.

The **inflammatory or noxious "soup"** consists of the host of chemicals that surround the nociceptor peripheral terminals in the tissue injury site:

- Chemicals released by **injured cells**: K^+, H^+, prostaglandin E_2 (PGE_2), ATP
- Chemicals released by **local cells** (mast cells, phagocytes, leukocytes, vascular endothelium, platelets): bradykinin, histamine, cytokines (such as interleukins and tumor necrosis factor α), serotonin, ATP, nerve growth factor
- Peptides released by the **nociceptors themselves** (the nociceptors are pseudo-unipolar bidirectional neurons that can release nuclear products at

both the peripheral as well as central terminals): substance P, calcitonin gene related peptide, cholecystokinin, glutamate

- Neurotransmitters released by **local autonomic nerves**: norepinephrine, epinephrine

Some of these act as direct nociceptor **activators** (e.g., K^+, H^+, ATP, bradykinin). These agents cause transduction at the peripheral nociceptor ion channel receptors. Others act as nociceptor **sensitizers** (e.g., PGE_2, nerve growth factor, bradykinin). These agents decrease the threshold of activation of the ion channel receptors on the nociceptor terminals. Thus, they increase the sensitivity of the pain detection mechanism at the peripheral level ("peripheral sensitization"; see below).

Peripheral sensitization refers to the increase in the sensitivity of the peripheral terminals of nociceptor neurons. It results in primary allodynia and primary hyperalgesia. The main mechanisms are as follows:

- Decreased threshold of activation of the transducer ion channel receptors present in the peripheral terminals of nociceptors, caused by:
  - Nociceptive sensitizer chemicals (see above) cause activation of protein kinase A and protein kinase C, resulting in posttranslational changes in the ion channel receptors. The decreased activation threshold of these modified receptors leads to increased transduction with noxious stimuli (primary hyperalgesia) and transduction with non-noxious stimuli (primary allodynia).
- Activation of previously "silent" or "sleeping" ion channel receptors by the nociceptive activators or sensitizers

An increase in transcription activity at the nucleus of the nociceptor neurons in the dorsal root ganglion in response to some of the nociceptive sensitizers (e.g., nerve growth factor, inflammatory mediators) leads to increased production, transport, and membrane insertion or release of (a) ion channel and other receptors and (b) neurotransmitters.

Central sensitization (6) is a very important phenomenon that refers to "an increase in synaptic strength in nociceptive circuits that results from synaptic facilitation or a reduction in inhibition" (1). It has been mostly studied in the dorsal horn of the spinal cord at the synapse between the first- and second-order neurons. It results in central amplification and facilitation of the synaptic transfer from the nociceptor central terminal (first-order neuron) to dorsal horn projection neurons (second-order neuron). It is an important mechanism for both inflammatory and neuropathic pain. It is responsible for secondary allodynia and secondary hyperalgesia, and it represents an important form of use-dependent neural plasticity. Central sensitization can be activity-dependent (i.e., depends on ongoing neural activity in the first-order neuron) and activity-independent. The initial (early; acute) phase of central sensitization is activity dependent and triggered by ongoing intense nociceptor input to the dorsal horn of spinal cord. It is the major role of the neurotransmitter glutamate, released by the central terminals of the nociceptor at the dorsal horn synapse. With this ongoing central input from the central terminals, the postsynaptic response becomes progressively stronger ("wind-up" phenomenon). The later (delayed; chronic) phase of central sensitization is transcription-dependent. Its basic mechanism involves upregulation of genetic activity (or removal of gene repression) in the nucleus of the second-order neurons, which leads to increased synthesis of proteins (receptors, ion channels, neurotransmitters, neuropeptides), which in turn results in increased synaptic efficiency and recruitment of normally non-noxious afferent inputs to elicit a noxious impulse, thus causing secondary allodynia and secondary hyperalgesia.

Mechanism of Preemptive Analgesia

Preemptive analgesia is the phenomenon whereby the need for postoperative analgesia is obviated ("preempted") by use of analgesic interventions before central sensitization is established. The basic idea is to prevent the establishment of central sensitization, as mentioned above (7). There has been controversy as to the meaning of preemptive analgesia. The one favored as a broad definition is that preemptive analgesia "prevents the establishment of central sensitization caused by incisional and inflammatory injuries (covers the period of surgery and the initial postoperative period)" (8, 9).

The mechanism of altered sensory processing of nociceptive input is complex and starts even before the first surgical incision (e.g., preoperative pain, fear, anxiety, and expectancy factors), continuing through the nociceptive processes involved in the surgical procedure (e.g., incision, tissue handling, retraction, etc.) and the early inflammatory changes following tissue trauma. Thus, proper preemptive analgesia ideally should cover the entire perioperative period. In this sense, there is a current tendency to talk in terms of perioperative "preventive analgesia" rather than the narrow earlier view of "pre-incisional" preemptive analgesia (10, 11).

Mechanism of Multimodal Analgesia

Pain mechanisms, as briefly reviewed above, are complex and multifactorial (12). The positive side of this is that pain may be targeted by different agents acting at different sites (periphery, nerve, dorsal horn of spinal cord, brain) or targeting different physiologic processes (transduction, conduction, transmission, perception, modulation). Using one single modality, however powerful, has its own limitations (e.g., reaching a ceiling effect, having unacceptable adverse effects [e.g., of opioids], etc.). Multimodal analgesia is an approach where different analgesics or analgesic adjuvants (e.g., opioids, acetaminophen, nonsteroidal anti-inflammatories [NSAIDs], alpha-2 adrenergic agonists, gabapentinoids) or different analgesic modalities (e.g., intravenous, local, regional, oral) are combined judiciously to obtain sufficient analgesia without unacceptable adverse effects. The basic idea behind multimodal (also called "balanced") analgesia is "achievement of sufficient analgesia due to additive or synergistic effects between different analgesics, with concomitant reduction of side effects, due to resulting lower doses of analgesics and differences in side-effect profiles" (13).

Multimodal analgesia can also help in preventing central sensitization and thus has some commonalities with the concept of preventive analgesia, although the primary focus of multimodal analgesia is on achieving sufficient analgesia by combining various analgesic agents or modalities (14). A large number of such combinations are possible, using various permutations of individual "elements" such as acetaminophen, NSAIDs, opioids, alpha-2 agonists, NMDA receptor antagonists, gabapentinoids, TRPV1 receptor agonists like capsaicin, and dual-action analgesics like tapentadol, and by also combining different modalities of analgesic delivery such as local applications of gels, creams, or patches, oral, intramuscular, intravenous, and regional anesthesia and blocks (15).

Conclusion

Pain is a universal phenomenon and can serve important physiologically adaptive purposes. The mechanism of such nociceptive pain includes transduction, conduction, transmission, perception, and modulation. However, in pathologic conditions such as inflammatory, neuropathic, and dysfunctional pain, additional complex mechanisms are recruited that make the nervous system more sensitized at both the peripheral and the central level. The idea behind preemptive (or preventive) analgesia is to minimize this sensitization process from setting in. Further, pain may be targeted by different agents acting at different sites (periphery, nerve, dorsal horn of spinal cord, brain) or targeting different physiologic processes. This is the idea behind using a combination of different modalities of pain management (multimodal analgesia).

References

1. Costigan M, Scholz J, Woolf CJ. Neuropathic pain: a maladaptive response of the nervous system to damage. *Annu Rev Neurosci* 2009;32:1–32.

2. Mitra S, Vadivelu N. Anatomy and physiology of pain. In Urman RD, Vadivelu N, eds. *Pocket Pain Medicine*. Philadelphia: Lippincott Williams & Wilkins, 2011, 2.1–2.5.

3. Basbaum AI, Bautista DM, Scherrer G, Julius D. Cellular and molecular mechanisms of pain. *Cell* 2009;139:267–284.

4. Mitra S, Vadivelu N. Mechanisms of acute and chronic pain. In Urman RD, Vadivelu N, eds. *Pocket Pain Medicine*. Philadelphia: Lippincott Williams & Wilkins, 2011, 3.1–3.5.

5. Vadivelu N, Whitney CJ, Sinatra RS. Pain pathways and acute pain processing. In Sinatra RS, de Leon-Casasola OA, Ginsberg B, Viscusi ER, eds. *Acute Pain Management*, 1st ed. New York: Cambridge University Press, 2009:3–20.

6. Woolf CJ. Central sensitization: Implications for the diagnosis and treatment of pain. *Pain* 2011;152(3 Suppl):S2–15.

7. Woolf CJ, Chong MS. Preemptive analgesia: treating postoperative pain by preventing the establishment of central sensitization. *Anesth Analg* 1993;77:362–379.

8. Kissin I. A call to reassess the clinical value of preventive (preemptive) analgesia. *Anesth Analg* 2011;113(5):977–978.

9. Kissin I. Preemptive analgesia. *Anesthesiology* 2000;93:1138–1143.

10. Dahl JB, Kehlet H. Preventive analgesia. *Curr Opin Anesthesiol* 2011;24:331–338.

11. Katz J, Clarke H, Seltzer Z. Preventive analgesia: Quo vadimus? *Anesth Analg* 2011;113:1242–1253.

12. Woolf CJ. Pain: moving from symptom control toward mechanism-specific pharmacologic management. *Ann Intern Med* 2004;140:441–451.

13. Kehlet H, Dahl JB. The value of "Multimodal" or "Balanced Analgesia" in postoperative pain treatment. *Anesth Analg* 1993;77:1048–1056.

14. Buvanendran A, Kroin JS. Multimodal analgesia for controlling acute postoperative pain. *Curr Opin Anesthesiol* 2009;22:588–593.

15. Young A, Buvanendran A. Recent advances in multimodal analgesia. *Anesthesiology Clin* 2012;30:91–100.

Chapter 3

Assessment of Pain

Juan P. Cata and Ehab Farag

Pain is defined as "an unpleasant sensory and emotional experience associated with actual or potential tissue damage, or described in terms of such damage." Recent governmental authorities mandate treatment of pain as a basic human right; moreover, they state that every patient has the right to assessment, treatment, and reassessment of pain, thus highlighting the important of adequate assessment of postoperative pain (1).

The assessment of postoperative pain involves gathering information from the patient through history and physical examination about intensity, location, characteristics, triggers, and factors that ameliorate pain. Because the pain experience has a subjective component, validated pain assessment tools are critical in appropriately assessing and treating pain.

Different clinical tools, including verbal, visual, and numeric scales and diagrams, have been developed to appropriately assess postoperative pain. Commonly, the history can be easily obtained since a surgical wound is the source of pain; however, some patients may have a history of chronic pain that may be confounded or even worsen after surgery. For instance, patients with chemotherapy-induced painful neuropathy often present for oncologic interventions far away from their neuropathic symptoms; for example, it may be seen in women who have received paclitaxel preoperatively and then present for unilateral or bilateral mastectomy. In other instances, obtaining a complete history and physical examination is difficult due to several barriers, including extreme age, psychiatric and neurologic disorders, and cultural differences.

This chapter describes why perioperative pain assessment is important and presents some of the clinical tools available for its appropriate assessment.

Why Is It Important to Assess Pain Preoperatively?

Preoperative modifiable and nonmodifiable patient factors may influence the development and perception of acute postoperative pain. Nonmodifiable preoperative factors include age, gender, ethnicity, genetic variants, cognitive function, and preoperative pain thresholds (2–4). In a study that included 1,736 patients, younger age was found to be associated with a higher risk (odds ratio [OR] = 1.3) for pain interventions early after surgery (5). Clinical studies demonstrate differences in pain ratings between males and females (6); however, those differences appear not to be clinically relevant in the context of postoperative pain. A study that included 14,988 patients demonstrated minimal difference in pain ratings among women and men within the first 4 postoperative days (7). Preoperative pain thresholds to different stimuli can also predict acute postoperative pain ratings. Several investigators have demonstrated that preoperative electrical and mechanical pain thresholds have the potential of predicting pain following surgery (8–10). The context in which a surgical procedure is performed may also predict postoperative pain. For instance, emergency surgery is a predictor for high opioid consumption in the postoperative anesthesia care unit (OR = 9.5, vs. no emergency surgery) (11).

Modifiable preoperative factors include smoking status, alcohol consumption, American Society of Anesthesiologists (ASA) physical status, preoperative pain, preoperative opioid consumption, patient expectations, anxiety, depression, and adaptive behaviors (2, 3, 12–19). A study that included 442 patients who underwent hernia repair surgery demonstrated that preoperative pain-related functional impairment intensity score, assessed using the Activity Assessment Scale (AAS) questionnaire, was a factor independently correlated with postoperative persistent pain (12). Preoperative distress and anxiety are important predictors of postsurgical acute and chronic pain (19, 20). The level of preoperative anxiety is different in patients with benign or malignant disease, thus the potential impact on the perception of postoperative pain (21). In a clinical study that included 101 women who underwent breast cancer surgery, preoperative distress predicted patients' experience of pain 1 week after surgery (22). Also, a recent study that analyzed data from 350 patients found that preoperative pain and preoperative opioid consumption predicted worse postoperative pain (3).

In summary, preoperative patient-related risk factors have been identified that have an effect on postoperative pain. Hence, clinical interventions targeted at improving or modifying those risk factors may improve postoperative pain management.

How and Why Is It Important to Assess Pain Intraoperatively?

Assessing pain intraoperatively can be particularly challenging even to the most experienced anesthesia practitioner because general anesthesia remains the most commonly used anesthesia technique. More importantly, the use of general anesthesia has been associated with significantly worse postoperative pain (OR = 3.96 vs. regional anesthesia) (23).

Since verbal communication is not feasible in patients under general anesthesia, anesthesia practitioners have to rely on clinical signs and information obtained from monitoring to assess intraoperative pain. Clinical signs obtained from physical examination include a rise in systemic blood pressure, tachycardia, grimacing, tearing, movement or extremity withdrawal, and/or sweating. Unfortunately, relying on these signs may be unspecific (24). The clinical scenario is different in patients undergoing surgery under regional anesthesia since they may remain fully awake or mildly sedated and communicative; hence, intraoperative pain monitoring is easier. A caveat is when deep levels of sedation are used as an adjunct to regional anesthesia.

In recent years anesthesia practitioners have tried to monitor intraoperative pain by analyzing parameters obtained from electroencephalography, electromyography, or somatosensory evoked potentials (25–27). A recent study indicates a possible association between state entropy and early postoperative pain (26). Moreover, the use of spectral edge frequency (SEF) has been positively correlated with postoperative pain. Gurman and colleagues demonstrated that maintaining the SEF between 8 and 12 Hz for at least 80% of the anesthetic time was associated with a lower visual analog scale (VAS) pain score after surgery. Although the difference in pain scores between patients maintained between SEF 8 and 12 Hz and those who remained outside that range was statistically significant, the clinical relevance is not that impressive, since the actual difference was only 0.6 points on the VAS (28). The bispectral index is not sensitive for intraoperative pain monitoring; in contrast, the enhancement of the amplitude and the reduction in the latency of N20/P25 as well as P60/N70 potentials may be useful parameters to monitor the degree of intraoperative analgesia (25).

In summary, there are not objective methods to monitor intraoperative pain in patients under general anesthesia. More research is needed to investigate technologies that could facilitate intraoperative analgesia monitoring.

Why Is It Important to Assess Postoperative Pain?

Nearly one third of patients undergoing surgery complain of moderate to severe postoperative pain (29). Pain is associated with a cascade of physiologic events ranging from activation of the sympathetic system, modulation of the immune system, activation of peripheral and central neural pain centers, and activation of the hypothalamic-pituitary-adrenal axis. Thus, inappropriate pain assessment and therefore inadequate control of postoperative pain may result in an increased need for rescue interventions, myocardial ischemia, immunosuppression, persistent postoperative pain states, immobility, poor physiotherapy, and prolonged recovery. For instance, respiratory complications after thoracic surgery can be reduced with the use of regional anesthesia techniques to facilitate incentive spirometry. In this setting, a careful assessment of pain will include the use of pain scales not only at rest but also during coughing or deep inspiration, both of which are necessary for appropriate pulmonary function.

Postoperative pain assessment is not limited to the evaluation of the pain characteristics but should also include the efficacy of the analgesic interventions used. The excessive or irrational use of analgesics with the objective of easing postoperative pain can also be deleterious to the patient. For instance, the excessive use of opioids in the postoperative period is associated with unwanted effects such as respiratory depression, ileus, pruritus, sedation, and immunosuppression (30). On the other hand, the use of a high concentration of local anesthetics or adjuvant medications in the context of regional anesthesia is also associated with adverse effects, including motor weakness, cardiovascular instability, and urinary retention. Importantly, most of these complications are easily treated after conducting an appropriate history and physical examination. More recently, the phenomenon of opioid-induced hyperalgesia has been reported in patients receiving moderate to large doses of remifentanil. These patients usually report disproportionate pain scores after relative minor surgical interventions. An appropriate history and physical examination are essential in the diagnosis of this disorder (31). Finally, the intensity of postoperative acute pain appears to be associated with long-term pain-related outcomes: patients with higher pain scores within the first month after surgery have a higher chance of developing postoperative persistent pain (32).

Taken together, the clinical repercussions of inadequate postoperative pain management are several and detrimental in most cases. A careful assessment is indicated to appropriately evaluate and treat postoperative pain.

Pain Scales

Pain intensity in the perioperative period is typically assessed with use of one-dimensional scales such as the VAS, the four-point verbal rating scale, or the numeric rating scale; however, the postoperative quantification of pain is difficult since many psychological factors can influence pain. The three scales can be used to evaluate pain at rest or during motion, coughing, or deep inspiration. Of the three scales the verbal one has the least power to detect a difference in pain intensity. Perhaps the easiest to use in most patients is the numeric scale, which has numbers from 0 to 10 ("no pain" to "worst pain imaginable"). The VAS remains the most common tool for assessing pain in the perioperative period, and early investigations demonstrated that the relation between noxious stimuli and VAS score is exponential (33, 34). However, one-dimensional scales have not been recommended as the only tool for managing postoperative pain (35).

Multidimensional pain assessment tools such as the McGill Pain Questionnaire, the Overall Benefit of Analgesic Score, the Opioid-Related Symptom Distress Scale, the Brief Pain Inventory, and the modified Brief Pain Inventory exploratory have been used in the context of postoperative pain (36). Overall, these tools appear to perform better than one-dimensional scales in the assessment of perioperative pain.

In preschool-age or younger children who cannot comprehend the three previously described scales, pain scales depicting happy and unhappy faces have been used with success. Also, the observation of pain behaviors is extremely useful in children; crying, screaming, verbalizing, putting up physical resistance, and muscle rigidity can also be observed as manifestations of acute postoperative pain in children (37). Pain in elderly patients may also be difficult to assess due to fear of addiction, poor communicative skills, or dementia. Interestingly, pain scales depicting faces have been developed to assess pain in elderly patients (38).

Quantitative Sensory Testing

Quantitative sensory testing is a semi-objective noninvasive method of assessing different sensory modalities, including warm and cold perception threshold testing, heat pain, and cold pain detection threshold, mechanical, pressure, and vibration detection thresholds, allodynia, and dynamic wind-up (39, 40). Clinical investigation suggests that punctate hyperalgesia in the area of preoperative referred pain correlates with the severity of pain postoperatively, and only some of the elements of secondary hyperalgesia, but not those of primary hyperalgesia, correlate with ongoing pain (41). Also, the preoperative response to heat stimuli appears to be a predictor of postoperative acute pain after laparoscopic tubal ligation (42). Similar results were found in a study by Hsu and colleagues, who demonstrated that preoperative pressure pain tolerance and mechanical hyperalgesia significantly correlated with early postoperative VAS scores and morphine consumption after different types of gynecologic surgery (9, 43).

In short, quantitative sensory testing can be used in the preoperative period to predict postoperative pain and opioid consumption. Hence, it would help anesthesia practitioners identify patients who are at risk for higher postoperative pain scores and individual pain sensitivities. This could lead to the implementation of more aggressive perioperative analgesic regimens, specifically multimodal analgesic interventions in those at higher risk (25).

Conclusion

The assessment of pain in the perioperative period is key to the appropriate management of acute postoperative pain. The assessment should start in the preoperative period and should be continued during and after surgery. Several clinical tools are available, ranging from one-dimensional scales such as the VAS, the verbal rating scale, and the numeric rating scale, to multidimensional methods. The former are easier to use in the perioperative period but do not take into account factors such as analgesic side effects. The latter appear to be more sensitive for assessing postoperative pain and the efficacy of analgesics, but they may take longer to complete and are not applicable in patients with special needs.

References

1. Joint Commission. *Pain Assessment and Management: An Organizational Approach.* Library of Congress Catalog. Report no. 00-102701, 2000.

2. De Cosmo G, Congedo E, Lai C, Primieri P, Dottarelli A, Aceto P. Preoperative psychologic and demographic predictors of pain perception and tramadol consumption using intravenous patient-controlled analgesia. *Clin J Pain* 2008;24(5): 399–405.

3. Kinjo S, Sands LP, Lim E, Paul S, Leung JM. Prediction of postoperative pain using path analysis in older patients. *J Anesth* 2008;26(1):1–8.

4. Klepstad P, Rakvag TT, Kaasa S, et al. The 118 A > G polymorphism in the human mu-opioid receptor gene may increase morphine requirements in patients with pain caused by malignant disease. *Acta Anaesth Scand* 2008;48(10):1232-1239.

5. Mei W, Seeling M, Franck M, et al. Independent risk factors for postoperative pain in need of intervention early after awakening from general anaesthesia. *Eur J Pain* 2008;14(2):149 e141–147.

6. Fillingim RB, King CD, Ribeiro-Dasilva MC, Rahim-Williams B, Riley JL, 3rd. Sex, gender, and pain: a review of recent clinical and experimental findings. *J Pain* 2008;10(5):447–485.

7. Schnabel A, Poepping DM, Gerss J, Zahn PK, Pogatzki-Zahn EM. Sex-related differences of patient-controlled epidural analgesia for postoperative pain. *Pain* 2008;153(1):238–244.

8. Buhagiar L, Cassar OA, Brincat MP, et al. Predictors of post-caesarean section pain and analgesic consumption. *J Anaesthesiol Clin Pharmacol* 2008;27(2):185–191.

9. Hsu YW, Somma J, Hung YC, Tsai PS, Yang CH, Chen CC. Predicting postoperative pain by preoperative pressure pain assessment. *Anesthesiology* 2008;103(3): 613–618.

11. Dahmani S, Dupont H, Mantz J, Desmonts JM, Keita H. Predictive factors of early morphine requirements in the post-anaesthesia care unit (PACU). *Br J Anaesth* 2008;87(3):385–389.

12. Aasvang EK, Gmaehle E, Hansen JB, et al. Predictive risk factors for persistent postherniotomy pain. *Anesthesiology* 2008;112(4):957–969.

13. Chang KY, Tsou MY, Chan KH, Sung CS, Chang WK. Factors affecting patient-controlled analgesia requirements. *J Formos Med Assoc* 2008;105(11):918–925.

14. Desai VN, Cheung EV. Postoperative pain associated with orthopedic shoulder and elbow surgery: a prospective study. *J Shoulder Elbow Surg* 2008;21(4): 441–450.

15. Donigan JA, Frisella WA, Haase D, Dolan L, Wolf B. Pre-operative and intra-operative factors related to shoulder arthroplasty outcomes. *Iowa Orthop J* 2008;29:60–66.

16. Granot M, Ferber SG. The roles of pain catastrophizing and anxiety in the prediction of postoperative pain intensity: a prospective study. *Clin J Pain* 2008;21(5):439–445.

17. Lautenbacher S, Huber C, Baum C, Rossaint R, Hochrein S, Heesen M. Attentional avoidance of negative experiences as predictor of postoperative pain ratings and consumption of analgesics: comparison with other psychological predictors. *Pain Med* 2008;12(4):645–653.

18. Shi Y, Weingarten TN, Mantilla CB, Hooten WM, Warner DO. Smoking and pain: pathophysiology and clinical implications. *Anesthesiology* 2008;113(4):977–992.

19. VanDenKerkhof EG, Hopman WM, Goldstein DH, et al. Impact of perioperative pain intensity, pain qualities, and opioid use on chronic pain after surgery: a prospective cohort study. *Regional Anesth Pain Med* 2008;37(1):19–27.

20. Scott LE, Clum GA, Peoples JB. Preoperative predictors of postoperative pain. *Pain* 2008;15(3):283–293.

20. Nielsen PR, Norgaard L, Rasmussen LS, Kehlet H. Prediction of post-operative pain by an electrical pain stimulus. *Acta Anaesth Scand* 2008;51(5):582–586.

21. Cassileth BR, Lusk EJ, Hutter R, Strouse TB, Brown LL. Concordance of depression and anxiety in patients with cancer. *Psychol Rep* 2008;54(2):588–590.

22. Montgomery GH, Schnur JB, Erblich J, Diefenbach MA, Bovbjerg DH. Presurgery psychological factors predict pain, nausea, and fatigue one week after breast cancer surgery. *J Pain Symptom Mgt* 2008;39(6):1043–1052.

23. Aubrun F, Valade N, Coriat P, Riou B. Predictive factors of severe postoperative pain in the postanesthesia care unit. *Anesth Analg* 2008;106(5):1535–1541.

24. Desborough JP. The stress response to trauma and surgery. *Br J Anaesth* 2008;85(1):109–117.

25. Coghill RC, Eisenach J. Individual differences in pain sensitivity: implications for treatment decisions. *Anesthesiology* 2008;98(6):1312–1314.

26. Law CJ, Sleight JW, Barnard JP, MacColl JN. The association between intraoperative electroencephalogram-based measures and pain severity in the post-anaesthesia care unit. *Anaesth Intens Care* 2008;39(5):875–880.

27. Sandin M, Thorn SE, Dahlqvist A, Wattwil L, Axelsson K, Wattwil M. Effects of pain stimulation on bispectral index, heart rate and blood pressure at different minimal alveolar concentration values of sevoflurane. *Acta Anaesth Scand* 2008;52(3):420–426.

28. Gurman GM, Popescu M, Weksler N, Steiner O, Avinoah E, Porath A. Influence of the cortical electrical activity level during general anaesthesia on the severity of immediate postoperative pain in the morbidly obese. *Acta Anaesth Scand* 2008;47(7):804–808.

29. Dolin SJ, Cashman JN, Bland JM. Effectiveness of acute postoperative pain management: I. Evidence from published data. *Br J Anaesth* 2008;89(3):409–423.

30. Aubrun F, Mazoit JX, Riou B. Postoperative intravenous morphine titration. *Br J Anaesth* 2008;108(2):193–201.

31. Lee M, Silverman SM, Hansen H, Patel VB, Manchikanti L. A comprehensive review of opioid-induced hyperalgesia. *Pain Physician* 2008;14(2):145–161.

32. Hickey OT, Burke SM, Hafeez P, Mudrakouski AL, Hayes ID, Shorten GD. Severity of acute pain after breast surgery is associated with the likelihood of subsequently developing persistent pain. *Clin J Pain* 2008;26(7):556–560.

33. Bodian CA, Freedman G, Hossain S, Eisenkraft JB, Beilin Y. The visual analog scale for pain: clinical significance in postoperative patients. *Anesthesiology* 2008;95(6):1356–1361.

34. Price DD, McGrath PA, Rafii A, Buckingham B. The validation of visual analogue scales as ratio scale measures for chronic and experimental pain. *Pain* 2008;17(1):45–56.

35. White PF, Kehlet H. Improving pain management: are we jumping from the frying pan into the fire? *Anesth Analg* 2008;105(1):10–12.

36. Chan MT, Wan AC, Gin T, Leslie K, Myles PS. Chronic postsurgical pain after nitrous oxide anesthesia. *Pain* 2008;152(11):2514–2520.

37. Blount RL, Loiselle KA. Behavioural assessment of pediatric pain. *Pain Res Manag* 2008;14(1):47-52.

38. Herr KA, Mobily PR, Kohout FJ, Wagenaar D. Evaluation of the Faces Pain Scale for use with the elderly. *Clin J Pain* 2008;14(1):29–38.

39. Backonja MM, Walk D, Edwards RR, et al. Quantitative sensory testing in measurement of neuropathic pain phenomena and other sensory abnormalities. *Clin J Pain* 2008;25(7):641–647.

40. Rolke R, Baron R, Maier C, et al. Quantitative sensory testing in the German Research Network on Neuropathic Pain (DFNS): standardized protocol and reference values. *Pain* 2008;123(3):231–243.

41. Gwilym SE, Oag HC, Tracey I, Carr AJ. Evidence that central sensitisation is present in patients with shoulder impingement syndrome and influences the outcome after surgery. *J Bone Joint Surg Br* 2008;93(4):498–502.

42. Rudin A, Wolner-Hanssen P, Hellbom M, Werner MU. Prediction of postoperative pain after a laparoscopic tubal ligation procedure. *Acta Anaesth Scand* 2008;52(7):938–945.

43. Brandsborg B, Dueholm M, Kehlet H, Jensen TS, Nikolajsen L. Mechanosensitivity before and after hysterectomy: a prospective study on the prediction of acute and chronic postoperative pain. *Br J Anaesth* 2008;107(6):940–947.

Chapter 4

Pharmacologic Agents: Opioids

Naum Shaparin, Atit Shah, and Karina Gritsenko

Introduction

When treating a patient in the perioperative period, the healthcare provider must consider the patient and any associated medical conditions the patient has, as this will influence the treatment plan. The practitioner must take into account the desired onset of pain relief, duration of treatment, and any potential side effects. Opioids are a class of medications used for pain control. By definition, opioids are any natural or synthetic drug with morphine-like properties. This chapter will discuss the basics of opioid use.

Background

Opioids are a class of medications that work through agonism of various receptors, including mu, kappa, delta, and sigma (1) (Table 4.1). These receptors are located predominantly in the central nervous system, but they exist peripherally as well. As seen throughout the body, these receptors are bound by substances that create both a desired effect, analgesia, as well as undesired side effects, including nausea, vomiting, constipation, and others as listed below (1, 2). Each receptor has a unique effect and side-effect profile, so it is important for the practitioner to understand the sequelae of each medication choice.

Table 4.1 Opioid Receptors and Their Respective Actions	
Receptor	**Action**
Mu1	Analgesia, urinary retention, bradycardia, hypothermia, euphoria
Mu2	Respiratory depression, bradycardia, dependence, euphoria, constipation
Delta	Bound by enkephalins, respiratory depression, dependence, constipation
Kappa	Analgesia, sedation, dysphoria, psychomimetic effects, inhibits ADH release
Sigma	Dysphoria, hypertonia, tachycardia, mydriasis

Pharmacokinetics and Pharmacodynamics

Each opioid is unique in its duration of action, period of onset, potency, and clearance. These factors become important when selecting an opioid to use for a specific patient.

Lipid Solubility

For example, lipid solubility can affect the onset of efficacy. Lipid-soluble agents provide a shorter onset time because they can pass through cell membranes more quickly and thus bind to receptors (3). Lipid solubility also allows the agent to be absorbed into fat more easily, which causes the drug to have a shorter duration of action. These characteristics allow fentanyl, a lipid-soluble opioid, to have both a quick onset and a short duration of action. The drug is taken up into fat through redistribution, so the analgesic effect is short-lived. In contrast, morphine, a less lipid-soluble opioid, has a longer onset time and a longer duration of action (3, 4).

Metabolism

The metabolism of each agent may also be important, especially in patients with comorbidities such as obstructive sleep apnea, where analgesia titration is essential perioperatively to avoid hypoxia/respiratory depression. Opioids are eliminated by a combination of biotransformation and excretion. Most opioids are metabolized in the liver and excreted by the kidneys. Kidney disease must not be overlooked when administering opioids, especially morphine or meperidine. These two medications have metabolites that are active and can build up in renal disease. These active metabolites can lead to prolonged sedation, respiratory depression, seizures, and even myoclonic activity (1, 3).

Remifentanil is the only opioid not affected by liver or kidney metabolism. Instead, it is metabolized by nonspecific plasma esterase in the blood. Breakdown occurs irrespective of liver function. This characteristic allows continuous infusions to run with an expected and reliable time to recovery. When turning off a remifentanil infusion, the clinician must consider titration of a longer-acting opioid to ensure adequate analgesia as the patient wakes up (1, 3).

Context-Sensitive Half-Life

When running an opioid infusion, the practitioner must also bear in mind the context-sensitive half-life of the various agents (Fig. 4.1). The context-sensitive half-life is the time it takes to reach 50% plasma concentration when an infusion is shut off. The context-sensitive half-life of fentanyl increases exponentially with time, therefore making it a worse candidate for infusions or sequential frequent bolus dosing. In contrast, remifentanil is so quickly metabolized due to ester hydrolysis that it has become a commonly used opioid during total intravenous anesthesia (TIVA) intraoperative anesthetics (1, 5, 6).

Opioid Dosing

Meticulous attention must be paid when administering opioids due to the potential for life-threatening side effects such as respiratory depression and sedation.

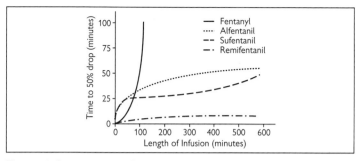

Figure 4.1 Context-sensitive half-time (time to 50% drop) as a function of length of infusion for commonly used opioids.

Table 4.2 Common Conversion of Opioids for Intravenous Use (in relation to 10 mg morphine)

Conversion Chart (in relation to 10 mg Morphine

Name	IV dose	PO dose	Duration	Half-life	Notes
Morphine	10 mg	30 mg	3–7 hr	1.5–2 hr	Parenteral morphine is 3x more potent than oral
Fentanyl	0.1 mg		1–2 hr	1.5–6 hr	
Sufentanil	0.01–0.02 mg				
Alfentanil	0.5–0.1 mg				
Remifentanil	75–100 mg				
Meperidine	130 mg	300 mg	2–4 hr	3–4 hr	
Codeine	100 mg	200 mg		3 hr	
Tramadol		120 mg			
Hydrocodone		30 mg	4–8 hr	3.5–4.5 hr	
Oxycodone		30 mg	4–6 hr		
Hydromorphone	1.5 mg	7.5 mg	4–5 hr	2–3 hr	
Methadone			4–6 hr	15–30 hr	

Table 4.3 Common Starting Dosing for Premedication, Induction, and Maintenance

	Premedication	Induction	Maintenance Bolus
Fentanyl	25–50 mcg	1.5–50 mcg/kg	25–100 mcg
Sufentanil	2.5–5 mcg	0.130 mcg/kg	5–20 mcg
Alfentanil	250–500 mcg	10–120 mcg/kg	250–500 mcg
Remifentanil		0.5–5 mcg/kg	25–50 mcg
Morphine			0.01–0.2 mg/kg
Hydromorphone			1–4 mg

Common dosing is given in references 1 and 7. Data from references 1, 3, and 5.

During the perioperative period, opioids are provided in serial doses and titrated based on symptoms. Doses are individualized for each patient, based on a combination of weight, previous opioid exposure (tolerance), comorbidities, and the severity of pain. The provider must be careful when administering opioids due to the varied patient responses: opioid-naïve patients should be given smaller dosages and opioid-tolerant patients may require larger doses. Opioids should always be titrated to effect.

In the acute postoperative pain period, goals of analgesia include providing pain control for acute triggers of pain (surgical stimulus). Typical starting dose regimens include morphine (1 mg q10–15 minutes) or hydromorphone (0.2 mg q10–15 minutes) in a monitored postoperative care unit (PACU). Alternatively, intravenous and epidural patient-controlled analgesia (PCA) dosing regimens can be used. In terms of pretreatment, morphine and hydromorphone have longer onset times and therefore may not be ideal for induction of anesthesia or for premedication. Short-acting agents such as fentanyl, sufentanil, and remifentanil are often preferred in the operating room setting; these choices would fall under the expertise of the anesthesia practitioner.

For patients who are opioid-tolerant, an acute-on-chronic-pain regimen would be calculated based on preoperative basal opioid requirements and additional medication for acute breakthrough pain, using conversion tables such as Tables 4.2 and 4.3. Additionally, the expertise of a pain medicine physician can be useful for the management of these more complicated patients.

Opioid Agonists

Table 4.4 lists common opioids, their predominant metabolites, primary route of elimination, primary method of metabolism, comments, and common routes of administration (1, 3, 5, 7–9).

Partial Agonists and Mixed Agonist–Antagonists

Nalbuphine is a partial agonist–antagonist. Nalbuphine affects both kappa and mu receptors. Benefits of a partial agonist include analgesia with a decrease in unwanted side effects, such as respiratory depression. Nalbuphine has been used to antagonize respiratory depression or pruritus caused by a full-agonist opioid. There is continued analgesia while antagonizing unwanted side effects (1).

Butorphanol is a partial agonist with activity on kappa and mu receptors. When given as the sole analgesic, butorphanol can cause respiratory depression; however, there is a ceiling effect that is lower than that caused by traditional opioids. In addition, studies have shown that patients receiving butorphanol PCAs have a lower risk of ileus compared to those receiving traditional opioids. Butorphanol can be given through intravenous, epidural, and transnasal routes (1).

Buprenorphine is a partial mu agonist with prolonged effects on the mu receptor. This makes it particularly difficult to antagonize with naloxone. Like butorphanol, buprenorphine also has a ceiling effect in terms of respiratory depression (1).

Table 4.4 Common Opioids, Their Metabolism and Routes of Administration

Opioid Agonist	Predominant Metabolites	Elimination	Metabolism	Route of Administration	Comments
Morphine	Morphine-3-glucuronide and morphine-6-glucoronide	Renal, biliary	Liver, GI tract	IV, PO, intrathecal, epidural, PR	Approximately 35% protein-bound. Buildup of morphine 6-glucoronide in renal failure patients leads to potent respiratory depression and narcosis.
Hydromorphone	Hydromorphone-3-glucuronide and hydromorphone-6-glucuronide	Renal	Liver	IV, IM, PO, SC	Metabolites do not have the clinical significance of morphine metabolites.
Fentanyl	Norfentanyl	Renal	Liver	IV, IM, transmucosal, intrathecal, epidural	Muscle rigidity can be seen with high doses. Has been associated with seizure-like activity on EEG.
Oxymorphone	Noroxymorphone	Urine, GI tract	Liver	PO	
Oxycodone	Noroxymorphone, oxymorphone, noroxycodone	Renal	Liver	PO	
Hydrocodone	Hydromorphone	Renal	Liver	PO	Formulations contain different amounts of acetaminophen.
Methadone	2-ethyl-1,5-dimethyl-3,3-diphenylpyrrolidine	Renal, GI tract	Liver	IV, IM, SC, PO	Mean termination half-life ~34 hours. Inactive metabolites
Codeine	Morphine, codeine-6-glucuronide	Renal	Liver	PO	Narcosis may occur in renal failure.

(Continued)

CHAPTER 4 **Pharmacologic Agents: Opioids**

Table 4.4 Continued

Opioid Agonist	Predominant Metabolites	Elimination	Metabolism	Route of Administration	Comments
Meperidine	Normeperidine	Renal	Liver	SC, IV, IM	Also possesses weak local anesthetic properties. Normeperidine has been associated with seizures, myoclonus, tremors. Useful for shivering.
Sufentanil	Desmethyl sufentanil	Renal	Liver	IV	Similar changes as fentanyl seen on EEG. Thienyl derivative of fentanyl
Alfentanil	Noralfentanil	Renal	Liver	IV	90–100% of patients given induction dose experienced chest wall, neck. and abdominal rigidity. Tetrazole derivative of fentanyl
Remifentanil	Remifentanil acid	Renal	Nonspecific esterase	IV	Ultra-short-acting so need transition drug to control analgesia

Opioid Antagonists

Naloxone is an opioid antagonist that works on the mu, kappa, and delta receptors. Clinicians must be careful when administering naloxone because in addition to reversing the respiratory depression, the analgesia associated with the mu receptor will also be reversed. In addition, the half-life of naloxone can be shorter than the half-life of the opioid administered, so repeated dosing or an infusion may be required. Other opioid antagonists include naltrexone and nalmefene (1, 5).

Systemic Effects of Opioids

Cardiac

Opioids can provide pain relief without causing much cardiovascular depression. These drugs can cause bradycardia secondary to stimulation of the vagus nerve. Unlike the other opioids, meperidine actually causes an increase in heart rate. This is due to the chemical structure of meperidine and its resemblance to atropine. In addition, morphine and meperidine may cause histamine release, which can cause a decrease in blood pressure (1, 5).

Respiratory

Opioids cause a decrease in respiratory rate. The patient's response to carbon dioxide is decreased while the apneic threshold is increased. Careful titration of opioids is mandatory to prevent respiratory depression/arrest, which can lead to cardiovascular compromise/collapse. In addition, opioids, if given in large enough doses, can cause chest wall rigidity, thus restricting ventilation. Neuromuscular blockade, if not contraindicated, can help in this situation, but proper airway ventilation must also be provided (1, 5).

Neurologic

Reductions in cerebral oxygen consumption, cerebral blood flow, and intracranial pressure are seen with the administration of opioids. There is minimal effect on the electroencephalogram (1, 4).

Nausea/Vomiting

There is a high incidence of nausea and vomiting with the use of opioids. It is thought to be caused by the medullary chemoreceptor trigger zone and can be treated with antiemetics. In addition, adjuvant medication can be added to the patient's pain regimen to decrease the opioid requirement. Adjuvants such as intravenous acetaminophen, ketorolac, and regional anesthesia are extremely effective in reducing the opioid requirement (1, 5).

Gastrointestinal

Opioids cause a decrease in gastrointestinal motility, with constipation being a common complaint. Patients receiving chronic opioid therapy typically become desensitized to many of the side effects associated with opioids, but constipation is a chronic complaint (1, 3).

Genitourinary

Urinary retention is a common side effect among patients receiving intravenous and spinal opioids. The urinary retention results from the urethral sphincter's inability to relax. The risk is greater in patients who have received spinal anesthesia. This side effect typically resolves on its own (1, 3, 5).

Endocrine

Opioids inhibit the release of catecholamines, antidiuretic hormone, and cortisol. Hemodynamics and volume status must be carefully monitored in these patients (1, 3).

Signs of Opioid Withdrawal

Opioid withdrawal occurs in patients who are taking large doses of opioids and have suddenly and dramatically reduced their intake, or patients who are addicted to opioids and have suddenly stopped taking them. Opioid withdrawal symptoms are outlined in Table 4.5. Symptoms can be divided into those seen early and those observed much later. Withdrawal from opioids can be extremely uncomfortable, but it is not life-threatening. Treatment from opioid withdrawal involves providing supportive care, but some medications can be given to alleviate some of the symptoms (1).

Use During Pregnancy

Opioids readily cross the placenta and are delivered to the fetus. Obstetric patients may have a fetus who is addicted to opioids upon delivery. The neonate may show signs of withdrawal 6 hours to 8 days after delivery. Opioid use during pregnancy increases the risk of complications to the fetus, such as preterm delivery and even miscarriage (1, 5).

Further Considerations for Postoperative Pain Control

When prescribing opioids for pain relief, clinicians should remember that opioid-naïve patients differ from opioid-tolerant patients. The former are typically

Table 4.5 Symptoms of Opioid Withdrawal	
Early	**Late**
agitation	abdominal cramps
anxiety	diarrhea
muscle ache	vomiting
tearing	nausea
runny nose	dilated pupils
yawning	
sweating	
insomnia	

sensitive to opioids, and the dose should be decreased accordingly. In the latter, the dose required to provide analgesia is often elevated (1, 7).

Conclusions

Opioids are a class of medications designed to provide analgesia. Like all other medications, there are desired effects along with unwanted side effects, and the practitioner must find the delicate balance necessary for each patient.

References

1. Barash PG, Cullen BF, Stoelting RK, Cahalan M. *Clinical Anesthesia*, 16th ed. Lippincott Williams & Wilkins, 2010:465–497.

2. Pasternak GW. Pharmacological mechanisms of opioid analgesics. *Clin Neuropharmacol* 1993;16:1.

3. Morgan GE, Mikhail MS, Murray MJ. Clinical Anesthesiology, 4th ed. McGraw-Hill Medical, 2007.

4. Bovill JG. Pharmacokinetics and pharmacodynamics of opioid agonists. *Anesth Pharmacol Rev* 1993;1:122.

5. Miller RD, Eriksson LI, Fleisher LA, Wiener-Kronish JP, Young WL. *Miller's Anesthesia*, 7th ed. Churchill Livingstone, 2010:769–823.

6. Egan TD, Lemmens HJ, Fiset P, et al. The pharmacokinetics of the new short-acting opioid remifentanil (GI87084B) in healthy adult male volunteers. *Anesthesiology* 1993;79:881.

7. Duke J. *Anesthesia Secrets*, 4th ed. Philadelphia: Mosby Inc., 2011.

8. Stoelting RK, Miller RD. *Basics of Anesthesia*, 5th ed. Philadelphia: Churchill Livingstone, 2007.

9 Scott JC, Cooke JE, Stanski DR. Electroencephalographic quantitation of opioid effect: Comparative pharmacodynamics of fentanyl and sufentanil. *Anesthesiology* 1991;74:34–42.

Chapter 5

Pharmacologic Agents: Non-Opioids

Yi Cai Isaac Tong and Sherif Costandi

Introduction

Effective perioperative analgesia has been shown to improve patient satisfaction, reduce length of hospital stay, and facilitate the rehabilitation process (1). The move toward a multimodal approach to pain has been shown to have many merits (2). It is thought that the use of non-opioids can facilitate the recovery process by improving pain management and reducing the opioid-related side effects such as nausea, vomiting, constipation, urinary retention, cardiorespiratory depression, pruritus, and sleep disturbances (3).

Non-opioids have three roles to play: they can serve as independent analgesics in the treatment of pain that is poorly responsive to opioids; they can be used to supplement and facilitate opioid analgesic use. This chapter focuses on commonly prescribed non-opioid drugs used in the management of perioperative pain. We review commonly used non-opioid drugs, their indications, and the evidence supporting their use in the preoperative, intraoperative, and postoperative settings.

Acetaminophen

Acetaminophen (paracetamol) is an antipyretic as well as an analgesic that acts centrally by inhibiting prostaglandin synthesis. In a placebo-controlled study, patients receiving paracetamol reported no difference in their pain when compared with placebo only in the first 6 hours after surgery, but the pain intensity was diminished in the paracetamol group from 12 to 24 hours (4). According to the results of a meta-analysis of randomized controlled trials, oral or intravenous acetaminophen combined with opioid had a significant morphine-sparing effect (5). In a comparison of side effects between the two groups, the paracetamol group had a significant decrease only in the incidence of vomiting, but patient satisfaction was greater (6). A possible explanation for the latter is the interaction of acetaminophen with serotonin 5-HT$_3$ receptors. The increase in serotonin is associated with a positive effect on the mood in addition to the decreased incidence of vomiting.

Adult oral acetaminophen, 600 to 1,000 mg qid, is effective as part of a multi-modal regimen and is well tolerated. The pediatric oral dosage ranges from 10 to 40 mg/kg, with a maximum daily dose of 60 mg/kg.

The injectable form of acetaminophen (IVA) allows its perioperative use when patients cannot tolerate oral medication. Results of a bioequivalence study indicated that 1 g paracetamol is equivalent to 2 g propacetamol, a prod-rug form of paracetamol. The recommended dosage of IVA for adults and adolescents weighing 50 kg or more is 1,000 mg every 6 hours or 650 mg every 4 hours, with a maximum single dose of 1 g, a minimum dosing interval of 4 hours, and a maximum daily dose of acetaminophen of 4,000 mg. The recommended dosage of IVA for adults and adolescents weighing less than 50 kg is 15 mg/kg every 6 hours or 12.5 mg/kg every 4 hours, with a maximum single dose of IVA of 15 mg/kg, a minimum dosing interval of 4 hours, and a maximum daily dose of acetaminophen of 75 mg/kg. Although the rectal route for acetaminophen delivery may be considered an alternative to IVA, rectal bioavailability can be poor, and absorption is delayed. Doses are usually 40 mg/kg.

Acetaminophen is almost entirely metabolized in the liver and excreted in the urine. IVA is contraindicated in patients with severe hepatic impairment, severe active liver disease, or a known allergy to acetaminophen. Acetaminophen should be used cautiously in patients with alcoholism, chronic malnutrition, severe hypovolemia, or severe renal impairment. Patients with severe renal impairment (creatinine clearance [CrCl] = 30 mL/min) require longer dosing intervals and a reduced total daily dose of acetaminophen.

Acetaminophen induces hepatotoxicity in chronic alcoholic patients, presenting with jaundice, coagulopathy, and abnormal aminotransferase levels. This seems to be due to either the induction by chronic alcohol intake of the cytochrome P450 system that converts acetaminophen to a toxic metabolite, or alcoholism-induced reduction in glutathione, responsible for conjugation with the toxic metabolites, thus normally preventing hepatotoxicity.

IVA may mask fever in patients treated for postsurgical pain due to its antipyretic effect and consequently may mask the signs of postoperative infection and sepsis. Acetaminophen has produced transient hypotension in critically ill patients with fever. The hypotension is usually mild to moderate but transient, within 15 to 30 minutes after the beginning of an infusion, and with maximal hypotension occurring between 1 and 2 hours after dosing. It has been attributed to the removal of the sympathetic drive associated with the fever.

IVA represents a major new approach to acute pain management in the perioperative setting. The lack of cardiovascular and hemorrhagic complications makes it an alluring option. It may be beneficial in reducing oral opiate requirements in patients susceptible to respiratory complications from opiates—for example, patients with obstructive sleep apnea, patients with increased intracranial pressure, morbidly obese patients, and pediatric and elderly populations.

Nonsteroidal Anti-inflammatory Drugs (NSAIDs)

NSAIDs are frequently used in the perioperative period as well as for the treatment of a variety of acute and chronic pain conditions. These medications act largely by inhibiting cyclooxygenase, which prevents the formation of inflammatory mediators, such as prostaglandins and thromboxanes. Two forms of cyclooxygenase enzymes (COX) have been isolated. COX-1 is present in all tissues, including the gastric mucosa, where it has a protective effect. COX-2 is an inducible enzyme and is produced primarily at the site of inflammation. NSAIDs' analgesic action appears to be related to inhibition of prostaglandin production both at the site of injury/inflammation and in the central nervous system (Fig. 5.1).

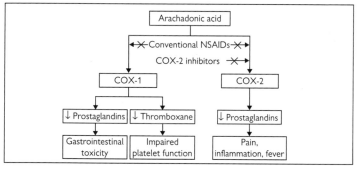

Figure 5.1 Mechanism of Action of NSAIDs.

Conventional NSAIDs, such as ibuprofen, block both forms of the COX enzymes. It was originally thought that selective COX-2 inhibitors would be associated with minimal systemic adverse events; however, COX-2 inhibitors have been associated with significant cardiac adverse events (7).

Ketorolac is a parenterally administered NSAID that is indicated for short-term (less than 5 days) management of pain. It is particularly useful in the immediate postoperative period. A standard dose (30 mg) of ketorolac provides analgesia equivalent to 6 to 12 mg of morphine but has a longer duration of action of 6 to 8 hours and lacks the respiratory depressant effect of morphine. The use of ketorolac as an opioid adjuvant has been studied widely. Cepeda and colleagues showed that adding ketorolac (30 mg IV) to an analgesic regimen for treating postoperative pain reduces morphine "rescue" dose requirements and opioid-related side effects in the early postoperative period (8). In a systemic review by De Oliveira Jr. and colleagues, several studies showed an overall effect of ketorolac in reducing postoperative nausea and vomiting (PONV). The number needed to treat or prevent one episode of PONV was 12.5. The review also showed evidence that the use of ketorolac decreased the time to hospital discharge in outpatient surgery populations (9, 10).

Ketorolac and other NSAIDs inhibit platelet aggregation and prolong bleeding time. Therefore, NSAIDs should be used with caution in patients at risk for postoperative hemorrhage (11). With long-term use, side effects are common. The most clinically relevant toxicities are related to the gastrointestinal, renal, hematologic, and hepatic systems. Dyspepsia, gastrointestinal bleeding, perforation, and ulcerations are all associated with NSAID use. Dyspepsia can be treated empirically with a histamine-2 receptor antagonist or a proton pump inhibitor. NSAIDs may also reduce renal blood flow and cause papillary necrosis and allergic nephritis. Aspirin (through COX inhibition) impairs platelet function for the life of the platelet (7–10 days). Patients with asthma have an increased incidence of aspirin sensitivity, particularly if they have a history of nasal polyps. NSAIDs can precipitate a potentially life-threatening exacerbation of reactive airway disease in patients with aspirin-induced asthma.

In summary, NSAIDs have a role in both acute and chronic pain. Their use in the perioperative setting may prove beneficial to patients. NSAIDs may not only supplement opioids but may also decrease the incidence of opioid-related side effects (Table 5.1).

Table 5.1 Non-Opioid Analgesic Dosing Information

Analgesic	Half-Life (h)	Onset (h)	Dose (mg)	Dosing Interval (h)	Maximum Daily Dosage (mg)
Salicylates					
Acetylsalicylic acid (aspirin)	2–3	0.5–1.0	500–1,000	4	3,600–6,000
Diflunisal (Dolobid)	8–12	1–2	500–1,000	8–12	1,500
π-Aminophenols					
Acetaminophen (Tylenol, others)	1–4	0.5	500–1,000	4	1,200–4,000
IV acetaminophen	2–4	5–10 min	650–1,000	4–6	1,200–4,000
Proprionic acids					
Ibuprofen (Motrin, others)	1.8–2.5	0.5	400	4–6	3,200
Naproxen (Naprosyn)	12–15	1	250–500	12	1,500
Indoles					
Ketorolac (Toradol)	4–6	0.5–1	10	4–6	40
COX-2 Inhibitors					
Celecoxib (Celebrex)	11	3	100–200	12	400

Gabapentin

Anticonvulsants have been found to be useful in many types of neuropathic pain conditions, such as trigeminal neuralgia, diabetic neuropathy, and complex regional pain syndrome. Gabapentin is unique in this class of drugs because it has been shown to be an effective adjuvant for postoperative pain (12). Gabapentin acts by blocking voltage-dependent calcium ion channels. This mode of action confers its antiepileptic, analgesic, and anxiolytic effects and blunts the development of hyperalgesia and central sensitization (13, 14).

While Gilron and colleagues reported that a 1.2-g dose of gabapentin given orally for 3 days was as effective as meloxicam 15 mg (15), Turan and colleagues showed that the same dose had similar effects to the COX-2 inhibitor rofecoxib (16).

In a systemic review of the perioperative use of gabapentin, Ho and colleagues noted that a single preoperative dose of gabapentin of 1,200 mg or less reduced pain intensity and opioid consumption for the first 24 hours after surgery. The time to first request for rescue analgesia was prolonged (17). As expected, the reduction in opioid consumption resulted in an associated decrease in opioid-related adverse effects. The incidence of postoperative vomiting and the incidence of pruritus were significantly lower in the gabapentin group (18).

The mechanism by which gabapentin modulates postoperative pain in the presence of opioids is currently unclear. It is thought that gabapentin and morphine may be synergistic due to their separate action on the peripheral and central nervous systems (19). Gabapentin may also decrease the postoperative morphine requirement by preventing the development of opioid tolerance (20).

Many studies noted that sedation was associated with perioperative administration of gabapentin. Ho and colleagues noted that the number needed to treat to result in one sedated patient was 8. No other serious adverse effects were observed with perioperative gabapentin use.

Ketamine

Ketamine, an N-methyl-D-aspartate (NMDA) antagonist, is widely used for the induction and maintenance of anesthesia. Ketamine has multiple effects throughout the central nervous system, including blocking polysynaptic reflexes in the spinal cord and inhibiting excitatory neurotransmitter effects in selected areas of the brain. Clinically, ketamine produces a dissociative state in which the patient appears "conscious" but is unable to process or respond to sensory input.

Ketamine has seen a recent resurgence of interest among providers as an adjunct in the multimodal approach to perioperative pain. Its ability to block NMDA receptors is thought to improve the efficacy of opioids and reduce the development of chronic pain syndromes. In a systemic review, Elia and colleagues noted that when ketamine was administered intravenously during anesthesia in adults, patients noted decreased postoperative pain intensity up to 48 hours, decreased cumulative 24-hour morphine consumption, and a delay to the time to first request of rescue analgesic (21). These results support the synergistic and additive effects of ketamine and opioids, believed to result from ketamine's NMDA blockade. One study followed patients after general anesthesia with intraoperative low-dose ketamine infusions and found that ketamine had beneficial effects on reducing painful sensations around the scar for up to 6 months after surgery (22).

Small doses of ketamine have been confirmed to reduce early postoperative pain and the development of chronic pain. A low-dose intraoperative ketamine infusion diminished opioid consumption and pain scores at 24 hours and

6 weeks postoperatively. Furthermore, a 24-hour low-dose ketamine infusion facilitated rehabilitation at 1 month and decreasing chronic pain at 6 months after joint replacement surgery (23).

While perioperative ketamine decreases opioid consumption, multiple trials looking at the change in opioid-related side effects showed no statistically significant difference between ketamine and control groups regarding PONV, pruritus, drowsiness, or urinary retention.

While ketamine produces intense analgesia, it also produces a myriad of effects on the body, including central sympathetic stimulation, inhibition of the reuptake of norepinephrine, bronchodilation, salivation, and cerebral vasodilatation. The risk of psychomimetic adverse effects such as hallucinations may be the cause of clinicians' reluctance to use ketamine. In several trials where patients received ketamine during general anesthesia after benzodiazepine premedication, 1.0% of patients experienced hallucinations with ketamine (24).

References

1. Rawal N. Postoperative pain treatment for ambulatory surgery. *Best Practice & Research Clinical Anaesthesiology* 2007;21(1):129–148.

2. Schug SA, Manopas A. Update on the role of non-opioids for postoperative pain treatment. *Best Practice & Research Clinical Anaesthesiology* 2007;21(1):15–30. doi:10.1016/j.bpa.2006.12.00

3. Rawlinson A, Kitchingham N, Hart C, McMahon G, Ling Ong S, Khanna A. Mechanisms of reducing postoperative pain, nausea and vomiting: a systematic review of current techniques. *Evidence-Based Medicine* 2012. doi:10.1136/ebmed-2011-100265

4. Cakan T, Inan N, Culhaoglu S, Bakkal K, Basar H. Intravenous paracetamol improves the quality of postoperative analgesia but does not decrease narcotic requirements. *J Neurosurg Anesthesiol* 2008;20(3):169–173.

5. McNicol ED, Tzortzopoulou A, Cepeda MS, et al. Single-dose intravenous paracetamol or propacetamol for prevention or treatment of postoperative pain: a systematic review and meta-analysis. *Br J Anaesth* 2011;106(6):764–775.

6. Gevirtz C. Acetaminophen: another tool for the treatment of postoperative pain. *Topics in Pain Management* 2012;27(8).

7. Wood AJJ, FitzGerald GA, Patrono C. The coxibs, selective inhibitors of cyclooxygenase-2. *N Engl J Med* 2001;345(6):433–442.

8. Cepeda MS, Miranda N, Diaz A, Silva C, Morales O. Comparison of morphine, ketorolac, and their combination for postoperative pain. *Anesthesiology* 2005;103(6):1225–1232.

9. De Oliveira GS Jr., Agarwal D, Benzon HT. Perioperative single-dose ketorolac to prevent postoperative pain. *Anesth Analg* 2012;114(2):424–433.

10. White PF, Raeder J, Kehlet H. Ketorolac: its role as part of a multimodal analgesic regimen. *Anesth Analg* 2012;114(2):250-254. doi:10.1213/ANE.0b013e31823cd524

11. Catella-Lawson F, Crofford LJ. Cyclooxygenase inhibition and thrombogenicity. *Am J Med* 2001;110(Suppl 3A):28S–32S.

12. Clarke H, Pereira S, Kennedy D, Gilron I, Katz J, Gollish J, Kay J. Gabapentin decreases morphine consumption and improves functional recovery following total knee arthroplasty. *Pain Res Mgt* 2009;14(3):217–222.

13. Gilron I, Orr E, Tu D, Mercer CD, Bond D. A randomized, double-blind, controlled trial of perioperative administration of gabapentin, meloxicam and their combination for spontaneous and movement-evoked pain after ambulatory laparoscopic cholecystectomy. *Anesth Analg* 2009;108(2):623–630.

14. Turan A, White PF, Karamanlioglu B, Memis D, Tasdogan M, Pamukçu Z, Yavuz E. Gabapentin: an alternative to the cyclooxygenase-2 inhibitors for perioperative pain management. *Anesth Analg* 2006;102(1):175–181.

15. Ho K-Y, Gan TJ, Habib AS. Gabapentin and postoperative pain—a systematic review of randomized controlled trials. *Pain* 2006;126(1-3):91–101.

16. Pandey CK, Priye S, Ambesh SP, Singh S, Singh U, Singh PK. Prophylactic gabapentin for prevention of postoperative nausea and vomiting in patients undergoing laparoscopic cholecystectomy: a randomized, double-blind, placebo-controlled study. *J Postgrad Med* 2006;52(2):97–100.

17. Matthews EA, Dickenson AH. A combination of gabapentin and morphine mediates enhanced inhibitory effects on dorsal horn neuronal responses in a rat model of neuropathy. *Anesthesiology* 2002;96(3):633.

18. Gilron I, Biederman J, Jhamandas K, Hong M. Gabapentin blocks and reverses antinociceptive morphine tolerance in the rat paw-pressure and tail-flick tests. *Anesthesiology* 2003;98(5):1288–1292.

19. Elia N, Tramèr MR. Ketamine and postoperative pain—a quantitative systematic review of randomised trials. *Pain* 2005;113(1-2):61–70.

20. Sen H, Sizlan A, Yanarates O, et al. Comparison of gabapentin and ketamine in acute and chronic pain after hysterectomy. *Anesth Analg* 2009;109(5): 1645–1650.

21. De Kock M, Lavand'homme P, Waterloos H. "Balanced analgesia" in the perioperative period: is there a place for ketamine? *Pain* 2001;92(3):373–380.

22. Laskowski K, Stirling A, McKay WP, Lim HJ. A systematic review of intravenous ketamine for postoperative analgesia. *Can J Anesth* 2011;58(10):911–923.

23. Guignard B, Coste C, Costes H, Sessler DI, Lebrault C, Morris W, Simonnet G, Chauvin M. Supplementing desflurane-remifentanil anesthesia with small-dose ketamine reduces perioperative opioid analgesic requirements. *Anesth Analg* 2002;95(1):103–108.

Chapter 6

Regional Anesthesia Techniques

Sherif Zaky, Maged Guirguis, and Travis Nickels

Introduction

Since the beginning of regional anesthesia more than a century ago, its practice advanced significantly (1, 2). It has been described as an art that requires a lot of experience and knowledge. A good understanding of anatomy is fundamental in performing any nerve block. Lack of knowledge about the anatomic variations of nerves and the surrounding structures can lead not only to failure of the block, but also to potentially serious complications.

Since the early attempts to block nerves to achieve either anesthesia or analgesia, different techniques have been described (2–4). Anatomic landmarks have been used to describe the locations of the nerves in relation to other anatomic structures that can be seen or palpated, frequently in relation to bony structures or arterial pulses. The subjective feel of pops or clicks has been described as an adjuvant to help identify anatomic layers.

However, since the results using anatomic landmarks were not great, nerve stimulation was then employed to help direct the needle toward the targeted nerve. The combination of anatomic landmarks plus the use of nerve stimulation led to a significant improvement in success rates. However, even in the most experienced hands, there continued to be block failures that were unexplained.

Now, with the advent of ultrasound-guided nerve blocks, some of these cases of failure can be explained. We now know that nerve stimulation indicates proximity to nerves but does not guarantee the spread of the local anesthetic. The spread of the local anesthetic depends more on fascial layers. Even though many studies showed mixed results comparing ultrasound with stimulation, there is a trend toward the use of ultrasound in the most common nerve blocks (5). Debate continues as to whether stimulation used in conjunction with ultrasound is beneficial.

Most recently, continuous peripheral nerve catheters have shown to be very helpful for pain control in the postoperative period, especially for extended periods (6, 7). Furthermore, the postdischarge use of catheters is gaining popularity in the practice of regional anesthesia, but a special service should be established to follow these patients and ensure safety (8).

Available data indicate that regional anesthesia—both neuraxial and peripheral nerve blockade—does improve patient outcomes. Mortality outcomes are difficult to assess given the relative safety of general anesthesia; however, the largest meta-analysis (CORTRA) of randomized controlled trials comparing intraoperative neuraxial with general anesthesia demonstrated a statistically significant decrease in mortality with neuraxial techniques (9). Subsequent studies (10, 11), however, have shown mixed results, leading to some controversy and inconsistent evidence for the reduction of mortality with epidural analgesia. Evidence is stronger that regional anesthesia may improve cardiac (12), pulmonary (13), and gastrointestinal (14) outcomes. Most convincingly, recent meta-analyses (15, 16) demonstrate that both epidural and continuous peripheral nerve blocks provide superior pain control compared to systemic opioids; this is a particularly important outcome given the recent emphasis on patient satisfaction and pain control as a metric for healthcare quality.

Upper Extremity Blocks

The nerve supply of the upper extremity originates mainly from the brachial plexus (Fig. 6.1). The brachial plexus is classically described as forming from the C5-T1 nerve roots, with variable contributions from C4 and T2 (17). In all, the brachial plexus travels through four distinct anatomic regions—interscalene, supraclavicular, infraclavicular, and axillary—and may be blocked in each region, depending on the specific indication. We will describe the most common upper extremity blocks, with emphasis on ultrasound-guided techniques.

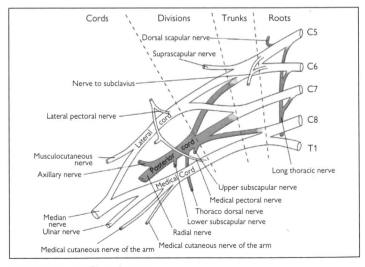

Figure 6.1 Lumbar Plexus Anatomy.

Interscalene Block

Indications

The interscalene block is best suited for procedures involving the shoulder (rotator cuff repair, arthroscopy, arthroplasty, etc.) and more proximal aspects of the arm. This block is directed at the root-to-trunk transition that occurs in the interscalene space, resulting in dense blockade of the superior and middle trunks (C5-C7) as well as components of the superficial cervical plexus, including the suprascapular nerve. Since block of the inferior trunk (C8-T1) is often poor, the interscalene approach is not usually indicated for forearm or hand surgery (18).

Ultrasound-Guided Technique

1. The patient is placed in a supine or semisitting position with the head facing away from the side to be blocked.
2. At the level of the cricoid cartilage, the probe is oriented in the transverse plane to identify the carotid artery. The plexus will appear as a column of hypoechoic nodules between the anterior and middle scalene muscles.
3. After the skin and subcutaneous tissue is infiltrated with local anesthesia, the block needle is then inserted in plane toward the plexus, typically in a lateral-to-medial direction.
4. The needle is advanced until it lies between the superior and middle trunks of the plexus.
5. After aspiration to rule out intravascular needle placement, a total of 15 to 20 mL of local anesthetic is injected while observing ultrasound spread.

Complications

Due to the proximity of the phrenic nerve, ipsilateral diaphragm paralysis occurs in nearly 100% of cases and may result in shortness of breath and even respiratory failure in those with respiratory insufficiency or contralateral phrenic nerve compromise (19). Horner's syndrome from blockade of the sympathetic chain occurs in the majority of cases as well, resulting in mydriasis, ptosis, and anhydrosis of the ipsilateral side. Further, blockade of the recurrent laryngeal nerve, although much more rare, may lead to hoarseness and even complete airway obstruction in those with contralateral vocal cord palsy (20). More serious complications consist of intrathecal injection and total spinal, pneumothorax, and vascular injury/injection.

Supraclavicular Block

Indications

The supraclavicular block is indicated for open or arthroscopic procedures of the arm, elbow, or forearm. This block targets the trunk-to-division transition that occurs at the level of the supraclavicular fossa (21).

Ultrasound Guinded Technique

1. The patient is placed in a supine or semisitting position with the head facing away from the side to be blocked.
2. The transducer is positioned in the transverse plane just cephalad to the clavicle at its midpoint.

3. The supraclavicular fossa is then scanned to obtain a cross-sectional view of the subclavian artery, which lies above the first rib. Superolateral to the artery, the plexus will appear as hyperechoic round structures with the appearance of a bunch of grapes.
4. After local infiltration of the skin, the block needle is then inserted in plane toward the plexus in a lateral-to-medial direction.
5. After heme-negative aspiration, 15 to 25 mL of local anesthetic is injected around the plexus while confirming ultrasound spread. This approach is amenable to continuous catheter placement as well.

Complications

Pneumothorax is the most common serious complication of the supraclavicular block, given the proximity to the cervical pleura, almost necessitating ultrasound guidance. Vascular injury, Horner's syndrome, recurrent laryngeal nerve paralysis, and phrenic nerve paralysis (22) occur as well, but less often than with the interscalene block.

Infraclavicular Block

Indications

The infraclavicular block is applied at the level of the three cords and is best suited for procedures involving the distal humerus, elbow, forearm, and hand. Blockade at this level negates the need for separate blocks of the musculocutaneous nerve, an advantage over the axillary approach.

Ultrasound Guided Technique

1. With the patient in the supine or semisitting position, the transducer is placed just inferior to the clavicle in a parasagittal position, medial to the coracoid process.
2. Attempts are made to visualize the axillary artery (typically 3–5 cm deep) and the surrounding hyperechoic cords of the brachial plexus.
3. After local infiltration of the skin, the block needle is advanced from the cephalad aspect along the plane of the probe.
4. The needle is initially directed toward the posterior aspect of the axillary artery. Once reached, 20 to 30 mL of local anesthetic is injected following careful aspiration. This should result in cephalad and caudad spread of anesthetic around the artery, yielding a donut-shaped lucent ring.

Complications

Vascular injury is the most serious complication, considering the depth of the vessels and difficulty with external compression. This block might be more painful to the patient than other upper extremity blocks due to the depth of the needle path.

Axillary Block

Indications

Performed at the level of the terminal branches in the axilla, the axillary block is indicated for procedures of the forearm and hand. In contrast to the more proximal approaches, care must be taken to specifically target the musculocutaneous nerve, which lies outside of the axillary sheath. Further, if a tourniquet is employed, the intercostobrachial nerve (T1–2) must also be blocked using ring infiltration of the proximal axilla.

Ultrasound-Guided Technique

1. The patient is positioned with the shoulder abducted and elbow flexed.
2. The probe is positioned high in the axilla—perpendicular to the long axis of the arm—to identify the pulsating axillary artery.
3. Attempts are then made to visualize the hyperechoic median, radial, and ulnar nerves surrounding the artery. The musculocutaneous nerve is typically found approximately 3 cm lateral to the rest of the bundle between the coracobrachialis and biceps muscles.
4. Once the nerves are identified, the needle is inserted in plane and directed toward each of the four nerves. Local anesthetic is injected, again after heme-negative aspiration, until circumferential spread is achieved for each (typically 5–7 mL per nerve).

Complications

While the overall safety margin of this block is high, vascular puncture, intravascular injection, and peripheral nerve injury may result.

Lower Extremity Blocks

The nerve supply of the lower extremity is derived from both the lumbar (L1-L4) and sacral (L4-S4) plexuses. Thus, in contrast to the upper extremity, at least two peripheral nerve blocks are needed to provide anesthesia or analgesia to the entire lower limb. The lumbar plexus lies within the psoas major muscle and gives rise to several terminal branches that are of interest to lower extremity nerve blockade (Fig. 6.2). The sacral plexus forms mainly the sciatic nerve and other small cutaneous branches.

A wide variety of blocks and approaches are available for lower extremity anesthesia and analgesia. The following, with particular attention to ultrasound-guided techniques, are the most commonly employed in clinical practice.

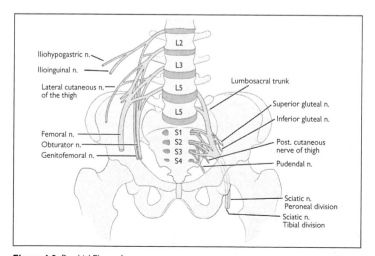

Figure 6.2 Brachial Plexus Anatomy.

Femoral Nerve Block

Indications

This block is indicated as the primary anesthetic in very few procedures involving the anterior thigh (e.g., repair of quadriceps tendon and patellar fractures) but finds great utility in postoperative pain control after femur and knee surgery, especially total knee arthroplasty (23). When combined with blockade of the sciatic nerve, complete anesthesia below the mid-thigh is achieved.

Ultrasound Guided Technique

1. The patient is placed in the supine position with the bed flattened.
2. The transducer is placed below the inguinal crease and the femoral artery is visualized. The femoral nerve lies approximately 1 to 2 cm lateral to the artery, on top of the iliacus muscle and deep to the fascia lata and fascia iliaca.
3. Once the nerve is identified and local anesthesia of the skin is achieved, the needle is advanced in plane in a lateral-to-medial direction toward the femoral nerve.
4. When the needle tip is visualized adjacent to the nerve under the fascia iliaca, approximately 20 mL of local anesthetic is injected after careful aspiration. Needle repositioning may be required to ensure adequate spread around the nerve.
5. A continuous catheter is frequently employed for postoperative pain control using a Tuohy needle.

Complications

As with all peripheral nerve blocks, intravascular injection, nerve damage, and hematoma formation are possible; however, these risks are minimal with ultrasound guidance and further mitigated by the superficial location of the structures and ease of compressibility.

Sciatic Nerve Block

Indications

Generally used in combination with a femoral nerve block, this block is indicated for foot and ankle surgery and also for postoperative analgesia following knee surgery.

Classic (Labat) Technique

1. The patient is positioned with the operative side up in the lateral decubitus position, tilted slightly forward. The operative leg is flexed with the foot resting on the dependent leg.
2. The surgeon palpates and marks the greater trochanter and the posterior superior iliac spine (PSIS), and then draws a line connecting the PSIS and the greater trochanter.
3. A perpendicular line is drawn bisecting this line and extending 5 cm caudad.
4. A 10-cm stimulating needle is advanced after local infiltration of the skin. As the needle is advanced, stimulation of the sciatic nerve will result in twitches in the hamstring, calf, foot, or toes.
5. After negative aspiration for blood, approximately 20 mL of local anesthetic is injected.

Sciatic Block in the Popliteal Fossa

Indications

This block is best suited for foot and ankle procedures and is often combined with a saphenous nerve block if the surgery involves the medial aspect of the foot or if a calf tourniquet is used.

Ultrasound Guided Technique

1. With the patient positioned prone or lateral, the transducer is placed transversely in the popliteal crease and the popliteal artery is identified.
2. Posterolateral to the artery is the tibial nerve, which appears as a hyper-echoic circle with honeycombing. The common peroneal nerve is located lateral to the tibial nerve.
3. The surgeon scans proximally until the branch point of the sciatic nerve into the tibial and common peroneal nerves is identified.
4. After local infiltration, a block needle is inserted from the lateral aspect of the thigh in plane with the ultrasound probe toward the sciatic nerve.
5. Once the needle tip is adjacent to the nerve, approximately 20 mL of local anesthetic is injected following aspiration and confirmation of spread.

Complications

Complications are the same as for the sciatic nerve block.

Neuraxial Blocks

Central neuraxial blocks include spinal, epidural, combined spinal epidural, and caudal epidural injections. Each of these blocks can be achieved either with a single injection or through intermittent boluses or constant infusions delivered through a catheter. The main site of action for neuraxial blockade is the nerve root.

Indications for neuraxial blockade (24) include surgery of the lower abdominal, inguinal, urogenital, gynecologic, and rectal regions and the lower extremity, including orthopedic and vascular procedures. Use in obstetrics includes labor analgesia and surgical anesthesia for cesarean sections. Neuraxial blockade can be used to control pain after thoracic surgery, major abdominal surgery, and orthopaedic surgery (hip, knee), as well as for pain control after trauma (e.g., rib fractures) and chronic pain.

Absolute contraindications to neuraxial anesthesia (25) include patient refusal, elevated intracranial pressure, hypovolemia, coagulopathy, and local infection at the site of injection.

Relative contraindications include sepsis, an uncooperative patient, stenotic valvular heart lesions, severe spinal deformity, and a preexisting neurologic deficit. Table 6.1 gives information on neuraxial anesthesia in the anticoagulated patient (26), based on 2010 American Society of Regional Anesthesia and Pain Medicine (ASRA) guidelines.

The following anatomic landmarks are important when administering a neuraxial block (27):

• The spinal cord normally extends from the foramen magnum to the level of L1–2 in adults and L3 in children.

Table 6.1 Neuraxial Anesthesia in the Anticoagulated Patient

Thrombolytic Therapy	1. Patients scheduled to receive thrombolytic therapy: Avoid performing lumbar punctures and neuraxial anesthesia and avoid thrombolytic therapy for 10 days if these procedures have been performed.
	2. Patients who have received thrombolytic therapy: Do not perform spinal or epidural procedures.
	3. Patients who have received neuraxial blocks at or near the time of fibrinolytic and thrombolytic therapy: Neurologic monitoring q2h or less "for an appropriate interval."
	4. Patient with an epidural catheter who unexpectedly received thrombolytic therapy: There is no definite recommendation as to when to remove it. They suggest to measure fibrinogen levels (one of the last clotting factors to recover) for appropriate timing of catheter removal.
Unfractionated Heparin	1. For subcutaneous 5,000 U q12h prophylaxis, there is no contraindication to the use of neuraxial techniques. Epidural catheters should be removed just prior to the next dose of heparin and the dose delayed 2 hrs.
	2. For heparin 5,000 U sc q8h or patients receiving >10,000 U daily, risks and benefits should be assessed on an individual basis.
	3. Patients receiving heparin for >4 days (heparin-induced thrombocytopenia) should have a platelet count before neuraxial block and catheter removal.
	4. With intraoperative IV heparin during some vascular surgeries:
	• Heparin administration should be delayed for 1 hr after needle placement
	• Remove catheter 2–4 hr after the last heparin dose; re-dose heparin 1 hr after catheter removal.
	• Monitor neurologic function postoperatively.
Low-Molecular-Weight Heparin (LMWH)	1. Preop LMWH should be held for 12 hrs prior to a neuraxial technique. With higher doses of LMWH, such as enoxaparin 1 mg/kg q12h, enoxaparin 1.5 mg/kg daily, or dalteparin 120 U/kg q12h, delay neuraxial technique for at least 24 hrs.
	2. Postop LMWH
	• *Twice-daily dosing.* First dose should be administered no earlier than 24 hrs postop. Catheters should be removed prior to initiation of LMWH thromboprophylaxis and the first dose should be delayed for 2 hrs after catheter removal.
	• *Single daily dosing.* First postop dose after 6–8 hours postop. Second postop dose after 24 hours after the first dose. Indwelling catheters removed after a minimum of 10–12 hrs from the last dose of LMWH. Subsequent doses should not be given for at least 2 hrs after catheter removal.
	• Presence of blood during needle or catheter placement does not necessitate postponement of surgery. In those cases the first dose of LMWH should be delayed for 24 hrs postop.

(Continued)

Table 6.1 (Continued)	
Oral Anticoagulants	1. Must be stopped 5 days prior to the planned procedure
	2. INR should be within the normal range for any neuraxial technique.
	3. Catheters should not be removed unless INR is <1.5 as warfarin therapy is initiated. Neurologic assessments may be continued for 24 hrs in certain instances.
	4. In patients with INR >1.5 but <3 the suggestion is to remove catheters with caution after reviewing medication records. It is also recommended to check neurologic status before catheter removal and continue checks until INR has stabilized at the desired prophylaxis level.
	5. In patients receiving low-dose warfarin therapy during epidural analgesia, the suggestion is to monitor INR daily.
Antiplatelet Medications	1. If taking ASA and NSAIDs only there is no added significant risk for the development of spinal hematoma.
	2. Ticlopidine (Ticlid) should be stopped 14 days prior to block.
	3. Clopidogrel (Plavix) should be stopped 7 days prior to block.
	4. Following administration, the time to normal platelet aggregation is 24–48 hrs for abciximab and 4–8 hrs for eptifibatide and tirofiban.
	5. GP IIb/IIIa antagonists are contraindicated within 4 weeks of surgery.
Direct Thrombin Inhibitors	ASRA recommends against use of neuraxial techniques in patients receiving these drugs (e.g. desirudin, lepirudin, bivalirudin, argatroban).
New Anticoagulants	1. Tricagrelor (BRILINTA): P2Y12 ADP receptor platelet inhibitor must be stopped 5 days prior to the planned procedure.
	2. Dabigatran (PRADAXA): Direct thrombin inhibitor. No official recommendation, but typically wait 2–3 half-lives to allow drug to be cleared.
	3. Prasugrel (EFFIENT): P2Y12 ADP receptor platelet inhibitor must be stopped 7–10 days prior to the planned procedure.

- In the cervical area, the first palpable spinous process is that of C2, but the most prominent one is that of C7.
- The spinous process of T7 is usually at the same level as the inferior angle of the scapulae.
- A line drawn between the highest points of both iliac crests usually crosses either the body of L4 or the L4-L5 interspace.
- The sacral hiatus is felt as a depression just above or between the gluteal clefts and above the coccyx.

Subarachnoid Block

Spinal anesthesia is also referred to as a spinal block or intrathecal injection. It blocks nerve roots as they course through the subarachnoid space. The spinal subarachnoid space extends from the foramen magnum to S2 in adults and S3 in children

Techniques

1. This block can be performed in both the sitting and the lateral position using either midline or paramedian approaches. In the sitting position, patients sit with their elbows resting on their thighs or a bedside table, or they can hug a pillow. In the lateral position, patients lie on their side with their knees flexed and pulled high against the abdomen or chest, assuming a "fetal position."

2. After sterile prep and draping, a skin wheal is raised at the level of the chosen interspaces with local anesthetic using a small (25-gauge) needle.

3. Using the *midline approach*, the spinal needle is placed with a slight cephalad angle of 10 to 15 degrees.

4. When the spinal needle goes though the dura mater, a "pop" is often appreciated. Once this pop is felt, the stylet should be removed from the introducer to check for flow of cerebrospinal fluid.

5. Using the *paramedian approach*, the needle is inserted 2 cm lateral and 1 cm inferior to the interspace and the lamina is contacted. After the bone is contacted, the needle should be walked off the lamina and into the subarachnoid space. An indwelling catheter can be placed for continuous spinal anesthesia (28).

Epidural Block

The epidural space is smaller than the subarachnoid space. It extends from the base of the skull to the sacral hiatus and surrounds the dura mater anteriorly, laterally, and posteriorly. The epidural space is bound posteriorly by the ligamentum flavum and laterally by the pedicles and the intervertebral foramina. Nerve roots travel in this space as they exit laterally through the foramen and course outward to become peripheral nerves.

Techniques

This block can be performed in both the sitting and lateral position using either the midline or paramedian approach. The prone position is often used in chronic pain management and is usually done under fluoroscopic guidance.

The classic approach is very similar to a spinal in terms of preparation and positioning; the difference is the use of an epidural needle (17 or 18 gauge, 3 or 3.5 inches long). Using the midline or paramedian approach detailed previously, the epidural needle courses from the skin just through the ligamentum flavum.

In epidural anesthesia the needle must stop short of piercing the dura. Two techniques make it possible to determine when the tip of the needle has entered the potential (epidural) space: the "loss of resistance" and "hanging drop" techniques.

The "loss of resistance" technique is based on the different densities of tissues as a needle is passed through the thickness of the ligamentum flavum into the epidural space. The needle is advanced through the subcutaneous tissues with the stylet in place until the interspinous ligament is entered, as noted by an increase in tissue resistance. The stylet is removed and a glass syringe filled with fluid or air is attached to the hub of the needle. Gentle attempts at injection are met with resistance and injection is not possible as the tip of the needle passes through the ligament millimeter by millimeter, with either continuous or rapidly repeating attempts at injection. As the tip of the needle just enters the epidural space there is a sudden loss of resistance and injection is easy.

The "hanging drop" technique is similar, but after removing the stylet, the hub of the needle is filled with solution so that a drop hangs from its outside opening. The needle is then slowly advanced deeper. As long as the tip of the needle remains within the ligamentous structures, the drop remains "hanging." However, as the tip of the needle enters the epidural space, it creates negative pressure and the drop of fluid is sucked into the needle (29).

Caudal Block

The caudal space is the sacral portion of the epidural space. The sacral canal is formed by the sacral vertebral foramina and is triangular. Each lateral wall presents four intervertebral foramina, through which the canal is contiguous with the pelvic and dorsal sacral foramina. The sacral canal contains the cauda equina and the spinal meninges. Near its midlevel the subarachnoid and subdural spaces cease to exist, and the lower sacral spinal roots and filum terminale pierce the arachnoid and dura maters. The sacral canal contains the epidural venous plexus, which generally terminates at S4 but which may continue more caudally. The remainder of the sacral canal is filled with adipose tissue.

Technique

1. The patient is placed in the lateral or prone position with one or both hips flexed, and the sacral hiatus is palpated.
2. After sterile skin preparation, a needle or intravenous catheter is advanced at a 45-degree angle cephalad until a pop is felt as the needle pierces the sacrococcygeal ligament. The angle of the needle is then flattened and advanced. Aspiration for blood and cerebrospinal fluid is performed, and, if negative, injection can proceed.
3. For adults, the block is often done with the patient in the prone jackknife position, but the lateral decubitus position or the knee–chest position may be used.

Truncal Blocks

Paravertebral Block

The paravertebral space extends from the cervical spine to the sacrum (30). It is a triangular space bounded anteriorly by the parietal pleura, posteriorly by the costotransverse ligament, medially by the posterolateral aspect of the vertebra and the intervertebral foramen, and laterally by the parietal pleura.

Recently, multiple studies showed that paravertebral blocks are as effective as epidural blocks for perioperative pain management without many of the side effects of neuraxial techniques. Some studies showed that these blocks may delay the recurrence of tumors and the development of metastases (31).

Indications

For preoperative pain management, a single block can be given in cases of limited inguinal hernia repair and minimally invasive cardiac surgery. Bilateral single blocks can be used for laparoscopic cholecystectomy, radical prostatectomy, and hysterectomy. A continuous paravertebral approach can be used for multiple rib fractures, major abdominal surgery, cardiac procedures, pelvic surgery, urologic procedures such as partial or complete nephrectomy, and open or laparoscopic surgery with a midline approach. Paravertebral blocks can also be used for anesthesia in cases of breast surgery, inguinal hernia repair, lithotripsy, and video-assisted thoracic surgery.

Techniques

1. The patient is positioned in most cases in the sitting position, but sometimes, as in trauma patients, these blocks are performed in the lateral position, similar to the position required for neuraxial anesthesia.

2. Three landmarks are important: the C7 spinous process, the lower border of the scapula (T7-T8), and the iliac crest (L4-L5) (32).

3. *Classic approach*: After sterile preparation and draping, skin markings are made 2.5 cm lateral to the midline at the levels to be blocked. These markings indicate the needle insertion sites and should lie over the transverse process of the vertebra; local anesthesia is used and the block needle is inserted perpendicular to the skin in all planes to contact the transverse process. When the transverse process is contacted, the distance between the skin and the transverse process is established; the needle is then withdrawn to the skin and reintroduced 1 cm beyond the transverse process at a 10- to 60-degree angle to walk off the transverse process superiorly or inferiorly. If during the positioning of the needle bone contact is established, the needle should be withdrawn to the skin and reoriented using a greater angle. As the loss of resistance technique to identify the paravertebral space is subtle, it should not be the only marker relied on. Instead, the skin–transverse process distance should be measured and the needle simply advanced 1 cm past the transverse process. After the injection is completed, either the process is repeated at another level, in the case of a single paravertebral block, or a paravertebral catheter is introduced in the paravertebral space, in the case of continuous paravertebral block (33).

4. *Ultrasound-guided approach*: described mainly in thoracic blocks using the same initial steps as the classic approach. A high-frequency transducer is used to obtain images in the axial (transverse) plane at the selected level, with the transducer positioned just lateral to the spinous process in the mediolateral orientation. Once the transverse processes and ribs are identified, the transducer is moved slightly caudad into the intercostal space between adjacent ribs. The paravertebral space appears as a wedge-shaped hypoechoic layer demarcated by the hyperechoic reflections of the pleura below (moves with respiration) and the internal intercostal membrane above (superficial). The needle is inserted into this space and local anesthetic is injected, resulting in downward displacement of the pleura. In a more commonly used technique, the scanning process starts 5 to 10 cm laterally with the probe in a cephalocaudal orientation to identify the rounded ribs and parietal pleura underneath. The transducer is then moved progressively more medially until transverse processes are identified as more "squared" structures and deeper to the ribs. Once the transverse processes are identified, a needle is inserted out of plane

to contact the transverse process and then walked off the transverse process 1 to 1.5 cm deeper to inject local anesthetic. The injection of the local anesthetic will result in displacement of the parietal pleura (34).

Transversus Abdominis Plane Block

This block provides effective analgesia when used as part of a multimodal analgesic regimen for a variety of abdominal procedures, including hernia repair, hysterectomy, cesarean delivery, and suprapubic prostatectomy. Within the transversus abdominis plane run the afferent nerve fibers of T6-L1 that provide sensation to the anterior and lateral abdominal wall.

Indications

This block can be used to provide postoperative analgesia for laparotomy, appendectomy, laparoscopic surgery, abdominoplasty, and cesarean delivery, and as an alternative to epidural anesthesia for operations on the abdominal wall, as in renal transplantation, abdominal wall reconstructive flaps, and inguinal lymphadenectomy.

Techniques

1. *Classic approach*: The patient is placed in the supine position. After sterile preparation and draping a 22-gauge needle is inserted via the lumbar triangle of Petit (the only area of the abdominal wall where the internal oblique muscle can be accessed directly), through two muscle fascias but avoiding any muscles on top of it. The triangle is formed posteriorly by the lateral border of the latissimus dorsi muscle and anteriorly by the posterior free border of the external oblique muscle, with the iliac crest as the base. The floor of the triangle from superficial to deep is formed by subcutaneous tissue, the internal oblique muscle, and the transversus abdominis muscle, respectively. The needle is then slowly advanced over the intermediate zone of the iliac crest until the definite "pop" is felt. A modified "two pop" technique using blind insertion of a regional anesthesia needle perpendicular to the skin, just superior to the iliac crest and behind the midaxillary line, also has been described (35).

2. *Ultrasound-guided approach:* Using the same initial steps as the classic approach, a linear probe is placed on the lateral abdominal wall cephalad to the iliac crest and caudal to the costal margin. After identification of the transversus abdominis plane between the internal oblique and transversus abdominis muscles, the needle is advanced through the different layers with a tactile feeling of a "pop" when crossing each fascial layer. Correct placement is identified by the solution separating the internal oblique muscle superficially from the transversus abdominis muscle (36). When a catheter is required, the space is dissected using 10 mL of saline or local anesthetic followed by catheter insertion for about 5 cm beyond the tip of the needle (37).

References

1. Koller K. Historical notes on the beginning of local anesthesia. *JAMA* 1928;90:1742–1743.

2. Matas R. Local and regional anesthesia: A retrospect and prospect. *Am J Surg* 1934;25:189–196.

3. McAuley J. The early development of local anesthesia. *Br Dent J* 1966;121:139–142.

4. Kovino B. One hundred years plus two of regional anesthesia. *Reg Anesth* 1986;11:105.

5. Liu SS, Zayas VM, Gordon MA, et al. A prospective, randomized, controlled trial comparing ultrasound versus nerve stimulator guidance for interscalene block for ambulatory shoulder surgery for postoperative neurological symptoms. *Anesth Analg* 2009;109:265–271.

6. Bauer M, Wang L, Onibonoje OK, et al. Continuous femoral nerve blocks: decreasing local anesthetic concentration to minimize quadriceps femoris weakness. *Anesthesiology* 2012;116(3):665–672.

7. Sripada R, Bowens C Jr. Regional anesthesia procedures for shoulder and upper arm surgery upper extremity update—2005 to present. *Int Anesthesiol Clin* 2012;50(1):26–46.

8. Abd-Elsayed AA, Seif J, Guirguis M, Zaky S, Mounir-Soliman L. Bilateral brachial plexus home going catheters after digital amputation for patient with upper extremity digital gangrene. *J Clin Med Res* 2011;3(6):325–327.

9. Rodgers A, Walker N, Schug S, et al: Reduction of postoperative mortality and morbidity with epidural or spinal anaesthesia: results from overview of randomised trials. *Br Med J* 2000;321:1493.

10. Rigg JR, Jamrozik K, Myles PS, et al. Epidural anaesthesia and analgesia and outcome of major surgery: a randomised trial. *Lancet* 2002;359:1276–1282.

11. Wu CL, Hurley RW, Anderson GF, et al. Effect of postoperative epidural analgesia on morbidity and mortality following surgery in Medicare patients. *Reg Anesth Pain Med* 2004;29:525–533.

12. Beattie WS, Badner NH, Choi P. Epidural analgesia reduces postoperative myocardial infarction: a meta-analysis. *Anesth Analg* 2001;93:853–858.

13. Ballantyne JC, Carr DB, deFerranti S, et al. The comparative effects of postoperative analgesic therapies on pulmonary outcome: cumulative meta-analyses of randomized, controlled trials. *Anesth Analg* 1998;86:598–612.

14. Marret E, Remy C, Bonnet F; Postoperative Pain Forum Group. Meta-analysis of epidural analgesia versus parenteral opioid analgesia after colorectal surgery. *Br J Surg* 2007;94(6):665–673.

15. Wu CL, Cohen SR, Richman JM, et al. Efficacy of postoperative patient-controlled and continuous infusion epidural analgesia versus intravenous patient-controlled analgesia with opioids: a meta-analysis. *Anesthesiology* 2005;103:1079–1088.

16. 16. Richman JM, Liu SS, Courpas G, et al. Does continuous peripheral nerve block provide superior pain control to opioids? A meta-analysis. *Anesth Analg* 2006;102:248–257.

17. Meier G, Buettner J. *Peripheral Regional Anesthesia: An Atlas of Anatomy and Techniques.* Stuttgart: Thieme Medical Publishers, 2007.

18. Orebaugh SL, Williams BA. Brachial plexus anatomy: normal and variant. *Scientific World Journal* 2009;9:300–312.

19. Urmey WF, Talts KH, Sharrock NE. One hundred percent incidence of hemi-diaphragmatic paresis associated with interscalene brachial plexus anesthesia as diagnosed by ultrasonography. *Anesth Analg* 1991;72:498–503.

20. Hashim MS, Shevde K. Dyspnea during interscalene block after recent coronary bypass surgery. *Anesth Analg* 1999;89:55–56.

21. Brown DL, Cahill DR, Bridenbaugh LD. Supraclavicular nerve block: anatomic analysis of a method to prevent pneumothorax. *Anesth Analg* 1993;76:530–534.

22. Guirguis M, Karroum R, Abd-Elsayed AA, Mounir-Soliman L. Acute respiratory distress following ultrasound-guided supraclavicular block. *Ochsner Journal* 2012;12:159–162.

23. Ng HP, Cheong KF, Lim A, Lim J, Puhaindran ME. Intraoperative single-shot "3-in-1" femoral nerve block with ropivacaine 0.25%, ropivacaine 0.5% or bupivacaine 0.25% provides comparable 48-hr analgesia after unilateral total knee replacement. *Can J Anaesth* 2001;11:1102–1108.

24. Warren DT, Liu SS. Neuraxial anesthesia. In Longnecker DE, et al., eds. *Anesthesiology.* New York: McGraw-Hill Medical, 2008.

25. Kleinman W, Mikhail M. Spinal, epidural, & caudal blocks. In Morgan GE, et al., eds. *Clinical Anesthesiology,* 4th ed. New York: Lange Medical Books, 2006.

26. Horlocker TT, Wedel DJ, Rowlingson JC, et al. Regional anesthesia in the patient receiving antithrombotic or thrombolytic therapy. American Society of Regional Anesthesia and Pain Medicine Evidence-Based Guidelines, 3rd ed. *Reg Anesth Pain Med* 2010;35:64–101.

27. Ellis H, Feldman S, Harrop-Griffiths W. *Anatomy for Anaesthetists,* 8th ed. Blackwell Publishing, 2004.

28. Brown DL. *Atlas of Regional Anesthesia,* 2nd ed. WB Saunders, 1999.

29. Kopacz DJ, Bainton BG. Combined spinal epidural anesthesia: a new "hanging drop." *Anesth Analg* 1996;82:433–434.

30. Karmakar MK. Thoracic paravertebral block. *Anesthesiology* 2001;95:771–780.

31. Boezaart AP, Lucas SD, Elliot CE. Paravertebral block: cervical, thoracic, lumbar, and sacral. *Curr Opin Anaesthesiol* 2009;22(5):637–643.

32. Finnerty O, Carney J, McDonnell JG. Trunk blocks for abdominal surgery. *Anaesthesia.* 2010;65(Suppl 1):76–83.

33. Hultman JL, Schuleman S, Sharp T, Gilbert TJ. Continuous thoracic paravertebral block. *J Cardiothorac Anesth* 1989;3:54.

34. Cowie B, McGlade D, Ivanusic J, Barrington MJ. Ultrasound-guided thoracic paravertebral blockade: a cadaveric study. *Anesth Analg* 2010;110(6):1735–1739.

35. Rafi AN. Abdominal field block: a new approach via the lumbar triangle. *Anaesthesia* 2001;56:1024–1026.

36. Tran TM, Ivanusic JJ, Hebbard P, Barrington MJ. Determination of spread of injectate after ultrasound-guided transversus abdominis plane block: a cadaveric study. *Br J Anaesth* 2009;102:123–127.

37. Hebbard P, Fujiwara Y, Shibata Y, Royse C. Ultrasound-guided transversus abdominis plane (TAP) block. *Anaesth Intensive Care* 2007;35:616–617.

Chapter 7

Medication Delivery Systems

Boleslav Kosharskyy, David B. Turk, and Karina Gritsenko

Introduction

Patient-controlled analgesia (PCA) is an innovative and relatively new method of pain management whose practicality and expediency have made it the preferred mode of pain management for moderate to severe pain (Fig. 7.1). Before the advent of PCA, a distressed patient relied on the vigilance of the healthcare providers for sufficient pain relief, and these needs often went distressingly unmet (1).

Multiple studies have demonstrated the superiority of PCA to conventional intravenous (IV) administration, with superior analgesic and adverse effect profiles. Its benefits include easier patient access to pain medication, reduced chance of medication error, and ease of titration to adjust to patient specifications (2) (Fig. 7.2). Compared with IV analgesia, PCA provides better pain control and results in greater patient satisfaction (2).

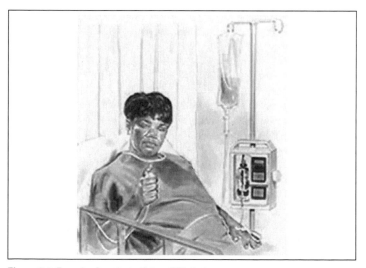

Figure 7.1 Example of a patient utilizing a PCA device.

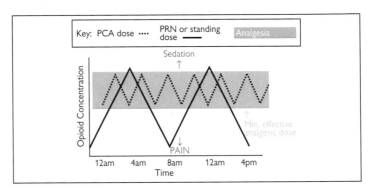

Key: PCA dose ····   PRN or standing dose ——   Analgesia

Figure 7.2 An illustration of patient-controlled analgesia (PCA) dosing. The PCA device permits for more frequent dosing of smaller increments, allowing the patient to avoid the peaks of oversedation and the troughs of break-through pain.

While traditionally many practitioners associate PCA infusion pumps with systemic IV opioid administration, they may be used to provide regional anesthesia, neuraxial anesthesia, and non-opioid adjunctive compounds. Patients with chronic pain syndromes who have failed to respond to traditional remedies may find relief from intrathecal infusion devices. This chapter explores medication delivery systems, compounds commonly used in analgesic infusions, and common template orders for their use.

Types of Infusion Devices

PCA can be considered a paradigm that allows for patients to self-administer analgesic medications. Speaking broadly, intradermal medications (e.g., fentanyl patch) or a 2-week prescription of oxycodone tablets could fit this broad definition. However, PCA commonly refers to a relatively new system involving the use of a sophisticated infusion device that provides small but potent infusions of medication to a patient, at his or her discretion, at set intervals.

The efficacy of PCA is based on studies that established that analgesia could be achieved and maintained by slowly titrating only slightly more medication than the minimum amount required to treat severe pain. The smallest plasma concentration at which pain was relieved was defined as the minimum effective analgesic concentration. By simply maintaining the minimum effective analgesic concentration with intermittent small boluses, effective analgesia could be maintained, while side effects of overmedication, such as sedation, could be largely avoided (3).

In the United States, PCA infusion pumps must pass strict safety standards and obtain U.S. Food & Drug Administration approval to be permitted for medical usage. Although pump models have evolved, they are all essentially programmable devices allowing the provider to dial in a discrete bolus dose, a lockout time between doses, a maximum allowable dose per unit time, and/or a background infusion rate, taking into account the type of device, the analgesic used, and the myriad characteristics of the patient receiving the infusion.

Current PCA infusion pumps may incorporate physical barriers to the burglary or misappropriation of the intravenous opioid; infusion bags or syringes

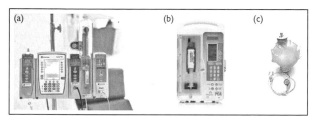

Figure 7.3 (a) Alaris PCA Containing Analgesic Medication Connected to Separate Infusion Pumps for Other Medications. (b) LifeCare PCA with Options for Locking and Safekeeping of the Opioid Medication. (c) Protable Braun disposable infusion pump that my be used for continuous intravenous analgesic regimens.

containing opioids are often literally behind lock and key. Other models may infuse local anesthetic medications, such as ropivacaine, into an affected part of the anatomy (e.g., a knee replacement). Such models may emphasize easy portability, so that the patient can wear the infusion pump by placing it in a small waist pack. Providers (physicians, nurses, allied health professionals) should consider whether the type of PCA pump selected is appropriate for the patient, taking into account his or her past medical history as well as past and present psychosocial phenomena (Fig. 7.3).

Pharmacologic Overview and Common IV-PCA Modes and Dosing Variables

Virtually any IV analgesic or anesthetic medication can theoretically be used for PCA purposes; practically, however, the choice of medication must be tailored to the patient's traits and needs. Opioids are the most frequently used agents in PCAs (Table 7.1).

Several non-opioid agents also have been employed for IV-PCA use. IV tramadol is used widely in Europe, where clinical studies have shown it to provide similar analgesic and patient satisfaction profiles. Tramadol acts at the central nervous system via several unique mechanisms of action; in addition to some mu-receptor binding, it also is believed to effect analgesia via interactions with serotonergic receptors and inhibition of monoamine reuptake, similar to tricyclic antidepressants (4). Although it is not available in the United States, clinical trials in Europe have shown that a demand dose of 10 mg tramadol is equianalgesic to 1 mg morphine; and demand doses of 10 to 20 mg with 5- to 10-minute

Table 7.1 Commonly Available IV Opioids

Mu agonists	Agonist–antagonists	Partial agonists
Morphine	Butorphanol	Buprenorphine
Fentanyl	Nalbuphine	
Fentanyl	Nalbuphine	
Meperidine		
Sufentanil		

Table 7.2 Guidelines for PCA Infusions

	Bolus dose (mg)	Lockout interval (min)	Continuous infusion (mg/hr)	4–hour limit (mg)
Morphine				
Adult	0.5–2.5	5–10	1–10	20–30
Pediatric	0.01–0.03 mg/kg (max 0.15 mg/kg/hr)	5–10	0.01–0.03 mg/kg/hr	
Hydromorphone				
Adult	0.05–0.25	5–10	0.003–0.005 mg/kg/hr	
Pediatric	0.003–0.005 mg/kg (max 0.02 mg/kg/hr)	5–10		
Meperidine	5–25	5–10	5–40	200–300
Fentanyl (mcg)				
Adult	10–20 mcg	4–10	0.5–1 mcg/kg/hr	
Pediatric	0.5–1 mcg/kg	5–10		
Sufentanil (mcg)	2–5 mcg	4–10	0.004–0.03	
Alfentanil	0.1–0.2 mg	5–8		
Methadone (1 mg/mL)	0.5–2.5 mg	8–20		
Oxymorphone	0.2–0.4 mg	8–10		
Agonist–Antagonists and Partial Agonists				
Buprenorphine (0.03 mg/mL)	0.03–0.1 mg	8–20		
Nalbuphine (1 mg/mL)	1–5 mg	5–15		
Pentazocine (10 mg/mL)	5–30 mg	5–15		

The provider may provide an intravenous bolus loading dose if necessary to establish initial analgesia. Individual patient requirements may vary; smaller doses are typically given to elderly or compromised patients. Continuous infusions are not recommended for opioid-naïve adult patients. Examples are PCA regimens that have been cited in the literature. Adapted from *Miller's Anesthesia*, 7th ed.

lockout periods have been employed (6). However, studies have shown that nausea and vomiting may be greater with tramadol than with morphine (7, 8).

In general, opioids are currently favored for IV-PCA usage; other drug classes are considered less efficacious for this purpose. Opioids are broadly defined by their actions at the mu receptor, being designated as either pure agonists, agonist–antagonists, or partial agonists. Despite variations in the patient population, some general guidelines for the administration of opioids are given in Table 7.2.

Agonists

Pure agonists are the most commonly administered compounds because they provide full mu-receptor binding, such that increasing the dose will result in linear increases in analgesia and allow treatment of moderate to severe pain. Dosing regimens are limited by a "clinical ceiling" of side effects that include increasing sedation, nausea/vomiting, and respiratory depression.

Mu agonists are equally effective at equianalgesic doses (10 mg morphine = 100 mg meperidine ≈ 2 mg hydromorphone ≈ 0.1 mg fentanyl). There are no major differences with regard to side effects; however, individual patients may experience nausea/vomiting or complain of pruritus with one agent but not another. A patient with allergies to morphine may very well tolerate a fentanyl PCA, while in other patients a fentanyl PCA may be less desirable because of its shorter duration of action. Thus, two opioids at equianalgesic doses may behave differently in the same patient and provide a very different experience for the patient. In addition, comorbidities may affect opioid choice. Patients with chronic renal failure may require a drug without active metabolites, such as hydromorphone, while patients with hepatic disease may require a shorter-acting agent that is not completely dependent on hepatic metabolism for its elimination, such as fentanyl.

Agonist–Antagonists

Agonist–antagonist opioids have a unique mechanism of action, namely kappa-receptor activation and mu-receptor antagonism. This striking difference results in an analgesic "ceiling effect," whereby increasing the dose does not substantially affect analgesia. These agents are therefore generally less efficacious in treating severe pain. Providers should exercise utmost caution when prescribing these compounds because they may precipitate an acute withdrawal syndrome in patients who are already receiving therapy with traditional mu agonists. Such patients should not be prescribed an agonist–antagonist such as buprenorphine (also known as Subutex, Suboxone, Norspan, etc., depending on the preparation) until a minimum time has passed (12–24 hours for short-acting opioids such as codeine but up to 3 days for longer-acting opioids such as methadone) and/or opioid withdrawal symptoms are clearly present (9).

Due to myriad factors, adjustment of analgesic therapy from traditional mu agonists to an agonist–antagonist should be coordinated in consultation with a pain specialist or provider certified to prescribe buprenorphine.

Partial Agonist

Mu partial agonists, such as buprenorphine, produce only a partial response in binding to mu receptors, which again limits the amount of analgesia that can be reliably provided. Therefore, similar to agonist–antagonists, they are not as frequently used in IV-PCA as mu agonists, but can be suitable for certain patients.

IV-PCA vs. Conventional IV Drug Administration

As mentioned above, IV-PCA is currently the favored mode of pain control: many patients prefer this method over the conventional PRN dosing schedules administered by the physician or nurse. Greater patient satisfaction may result from superior analgesia and/or perceived control over analgesic medications, bypassing the need to vocalize one's pain, request analgesic medications from hospital staff, and often impassively wait for its provision. One important factor in the decision to provide a PCA is to determine whether the patient can use the modality. The patient must be able to make decisions, understand how to use a PCA button, and reach, hold, and press the button. Issues such as fear, confusion, and other psychological phenomena may result in a patient accepting worse pain and being unable to obtain maximum benefit from the PCA. The decision to administer a bolus dose must be made by the patient and not by a nurse or family member, except for unique circumstances.

The incidence of adverse events from PCA does not differ significantly from PRN administration. There is a low rate of respiratory depression associated with PCA (<0.5%), and this does not appear to be greater than that associated with PRN or neuraxial opioid administration (10, 11). Risk factors associated with respiratory depression include use of a background infusion rate; concomitant use of a sedative or hypnotic agent; elderly, obese, or debilitated patients; head injury; hypovolemia; renal failure; and coexisting pulmonary disease such as sleep apnea (11–13).

Although better pain control and improved patient satisfaction are documented in PCA over conventional parenteral PRN analgesia, drawbacks of PCA may include hypothesized decreased cost-effectiveness, due in part to greater opioid usage by the patient (2). This increased cost is slightly offset by savings in nursing time; nevertheless, overall costs are estimated be as low as 1% of total perioperative costs and should not usually be taken into account when deciding whether PCA is appropriate for an individual. Patients using IV-PCA are also slightly more likely than those on conventional opioid therapies to experience pruritus with higher doses.

When prescribing IV-PCA, an order set should address any adverse issues that may arise. An auxiliary PRN medication should be ordered should the PCA fail to function, or should the patient report intolerable side effects from the selected medication. An order set should clearly document the therapy that the patient is receiving and should provide clear instructions to other healthcare staff. Table 7.3 lists the components of a typical order set.

Special Cases

Patients who have been using opioids chronically should be monitored more closely because their postoperative analgesic needs will be greater than those of the typical perioperative patient. Opioid-tolerant patients present with acute-on-chronic pain, and thus a baseline continuous PCA infusion may be needed to control pain in such patients; demand dosing schedules may not be sufficient.

Table 7.3 Prototypical Order Set for PCA		
Order Specifications	**Routine Monitoring**	**Instructions Provided**
Name, concentration, and dose of drug	Vital signs	Treatment of side effects (e.g., ondansetron for nausea)
Settings of device: demand dose, lockout interval, and continuous infusion rate (if applicable)	Analgesia or severity of pain Pain at rest/with activity	Parameters for triggering notification of the covering physician
Limits set (e.g., 1- and 4-hour limits)	Recorded amount of drug administered per set interval	Contact information (24 hours/7 days/week)
Supplemental and breakthrough medications	Use of breakthrough medication	Emergency analgesic treatment if PCA fails
Adapted from *Miller's Anesthesia*, Churchill Livingstone, 7th ed., 2009.		

Opioid-tolerant patients may also benefit from the addition of long-acting opiates, such as a transdermal fentanyl patch or extended-release opioids for basal opioid analgesic level. This technique, however, should not routinely be employed in opioid-naïve patients due to a delayed and slow onset of action and the potential for adverse effects such as overdose and respiratory depression.

Patients on chronic methadone therapy should be restarted on their oral methadone dose as soon as possible after surgery to meet basal pain needs; any additional postoperative analgesic requirements can be met via IV-PCA. These patients often require high doses and can usually receive them safely due to individualized opioid tolerance. Nonetheless, each patient must be treated as an individual, and the ability to tolerate higher doses does not preclude serious sequelae, such as respiratory depression.

Pediatric patients deserve special consideration because their analgesic regimens may differ significantly from those of adult patients; see Chapter 10 for more information.

If there are any concerns regarding pain management, a pain specialist should be consulted.

Intrathecal and Epidural PCA

The same concepts of PCA can be applied to neuraxial (intrathecal and epidural) pain management. Opioids, local anesthetics, or a combination of the two can be used because diffusion from the intrathecal and epidural space is typically slow, depending on the agent or combination used, and local anesthetic toxicity can be avoided. The use of opioids in neuraxial pain management plans is predicated on the knowledge that opioid receptors are present in the spinal cord; opioids placed in the epidural space can diffuse across the dura to gain access to receptors on the spinal cord. Intrathecal delivery is more common in long-term PCA devices for chronic pain but is used in some institutions. More common is the epidural method of neuraxial perioperative analgesia.

Epidural PCA

Epidural PCA or patient-controlled epidural analgesia (PCEA) is the second most frequently used and second most studied route of PCA acute pain management. PCEA optimizes analgesia by titrating analgesia to the patient's needs while minimizing side effects. PCEA may offer several advantages over a continuous epidural infusion, such as superior analgesia, greater patient satisfaction, and less epidural analgesic use. A meta-analysis comparing PCEA with continuous epidural infusions and IV-PCA found that for all types of surgery and pain assessments, all forms of epidural analgesia provided significantly superior analgesic profiles than IV-PCA. Continuous epidural infusions provided significantly better analgesia than PCEA; however, patients receiving continuous epidural infusions also had a significantly higher incidence of nausea/vomiting and motor block (14).

In contrast to IV-PCA, PCEA orders frequently incorporate a background continuous infusion rate to optimize potential physiologic benefits and maintain continuous neural blockade. Also, the use of neuraxial analgesia in and of itself can provide theoretically described benefits, such as decreased time to discharge from the postanesthesia care unit and less risk for deep venous thrombosis and pulmonary embolism. Meta-analyses have also shown intraoperative benefits, including decreased blood loss and a decreased likelihood for blood transfusion (15).

PCEA solutions are generally a combination of a local anesthetic (Table 7.4) and a lipid-soluble opioid (fentanyl or sufentanil), although other opioids (such as morphine and hydromorphone) have also frequently been used. In contrast to IV-PCA, optimal PCEA delivery variables (demand dose, lockout interval) are less definitive; there is also no standout choice of PCEA analgesic solution (Table 7.5).

It is important to consider the lipid solubility of agents used to assess the time course of the analgesia. In addition, the level of the epidural infusion effects can affect the risk of systemic side effects.

Perioperative epidural analgesia, especially with a combination opioid/local anesthetic-based solution, can decrease the pathophysiologic response to surgery and may be associated with a reduction in morbidity and mortality when compared to the use of IV opioid agents. It may also have a positive impact on pulmonary, gastrointestinal, and cardiovascular function (16, 17).

Table 7.4 Some Commonly Used Local Anesthetics
Lidocaine
Bupivacaine
Ropivacaine
2-Chloroprocaine
Mepivacaine
Prilocaine

Table 7.5 PCEA Regimens			
Analgesic Solution	**Continuous Rate (mL/hr)**	**Demand Dose (mL)**	**Lockout Interval (min)**
General Regimens			
0.05% bupivacaine + 4 mcg/mL fentanyl	4	2	10
0.0625% bupivacaine + 5 mcg fentanyl	4–6	3–4	10–15
0.1% bupivacaine + 5 mcg/mL fentanyl	6	2	10–15
0.2% ropivacaine + 5 mcg/mL fentanyl	5	2	20
Thoracic Surgery			
0.0625%–0.125% bupivacaine + 5 mcg/mL fentanyl	3–4	2–3	10–15
Lower Extremity Surgery			
0.0625%–0.125% bupivacaine + 5 mcg/mL fentanyl	4–6	3–4	10–15
0.125% levobupivacaine + 4 mcg/mL fentanyl	4	2	10
These regimens are samples from the literature; choice of infusion solution, rate, dose and interval may be institution-specific or adjusted per anesthesia practitioner. Adapted from *Miller's Anesthesia*, Churchill Livingstone, 7th ed., 2009.			

Concerns Regarding PCEA

The local anesthetics used in epidural analgesia may block nerve fibers of the sympathetic nervous system and contribute to **hypotension**. Vital signs should be routinely monitored for any patient on PCA or PCEA. Certainly, in high thoracic epidurals, there is a possibility of blocking cardiac accessory fibers, which can lead to both hypotension and bradycardia.

Motor block can result from use of local anesthetics in the analgesic solution, which may lead to pressure sores of the heels. Motor block usually resolves approximately 2 hours after stopping the epidural infusion; with prolonged motor block, the provider should evaluate the patient promptly for rare but significant adverse events, including spinal hematoma, spinal abscess, and intrathecal catheter migration.

Chronic anticoagulation is a concerning risk factor for **spinal hematoma**; epidural catheter removal must be coordinated with the anesthesia practitioner or pain specialist, who will recommend the earliest interval that anticoagulation can resume following removal (or, alternatively, how soon the epidural may be placed after anticoagulation therapy has been withheld).

Urinary retention, which may also result from IV opioid administration, is seen more commonly with intrathecal opioid therapies and results from opioid-mediated decreases in the detrusor muscle's strength of contraction as well as a decreased sensation of urge. IV agents that are more likely to cause decreased detrusor contraction include fentanyl and buprenorphine (18).

Pruritus is seen more commonly in patients receiving continuous epidural infusions but may manifest with PCEA therapy as well.

Intrathecal PCA

Studies have demonstrated the efficacy of intrathecally administered opioids for the long-term management of chronic pain, both cancer-related and non–cancer-related. The main reasons for consideration of the intrathecal route are inadequate pain relief with conservative medical therapy, intolerable side effects associated with oral/transdermal opioids, and/or failure of interventional or surgical techniques to address pain (19).

Implanted intrathecal infusion systems sidestep the blood–brain barrier, delivering medications directly into the intrathecal space. Currently, only two agents are approved by the U.S. Food & Drug Administration for this purpose, preservative-free morphine and the non-opioid peptide ziconotide, although additional agents and adjuvants have been used in clinical practice.

Patients who are noted to be responding poorly to conventional pain therapies may be referred to a pain specialist to determine whether they are suitable for this modality.

Summary

This chapter briefly touched upon PCA and PCEA. Healthcare providers can provide significant benefit to analgesic care by helping to coordinate the perioperative analgesic plan in concert with other providers from across the myriad disciplines.

References

1. Marks RM, Sachar EJ. Undertreatment of medical inpatients with narcotic analgesics. *Ann Intern Med* 1973;78:173–181.

2. Hudcova J, McNicol E, Quah C, et al. Patient controlled opioid analgesia versus conventional opioid analgesia for postoperative pain. *Cochrane Database Syst Rev 4*: CD003348, 2006.

3. Austin KL, Stapleton JV, Mather LE. Relationship between blood meperidine concentrations and analgesic response: a preliminary report. *Anesthesiology* 1980;53:460–466.

4. Bamigbade TA, Davidson C, et al. Actions of tramadol, its enantiomers and principal metabolite, O-desmethyltramadol, on serotonin (5-HT) efflux and uptake in the rat dorsal raphe nucleus. *Br J Anaesth* 1997;79:352–356.

5. Grass JA. Patient-controlled analgesia. *Anesth Analg* 2005;101:S44–S61.

6. Ng KF, Tsui SL, Yang JC, Ho ET. Increased nausea and dizziness when using tramadol for post-operative patient controlled analgesia compared with morphine after intraoperative loading with morphine. *Eur J Anaesthesiol* 1998;15(5):565–570.

7. Silvasti M, Svartling N, Pitkanen M, Rosenberg PH. Comparison of intravenous patient-controlled analgesia with tramadol versus morphine after microvascular breast reconstruction. *Eur J Anaesthesiol* 2000;17(7):448–455.

8. National Alliance of Advocates for Buprenorphine Treatment. *What is Precipitated Withdrawal?* Available at: http://www.naabt.org/documents/naabt_precipwd.pdf

9. Looi-Lyons LC, Chung FF, Chan VW, et al. Respiratory depression: An adverse outcome during patient-controlled analgesia therapy. *J Clin Anesth* 1996;8:151.

10. Etches RC. Respiratory depression associated with patient-controlled analgesia: A review of eight cases. *Can J Anaesth* 1994;41:125.

11. Baxter AD. Respiratory depression with patient-controlled analgesia. *Can J Anesth* 1994;41:87–90.

12. Baird MB, Schug SA. Safety aspects of postoperative pain relief. *Pain Digest* 1996;6:219–225.

13. Wu CL, Cohen SR, Richman JM, et al. Efficacy of postoperative patient-controlled and continuous infusion epidural analgesia versus intravenous patient-controlled analgesia with opioids: A meta-analysis. *Anesthesiology* 2005;103:1079.

14. Mauermann WJ, Shilling AM, Zhiyi Z. A comparison of neuraxial block versus general anesthesia for elective total hip replacement: A meta-analysis. *Regional Anesthesia* 2006;103(4).

15. Liu S, Carpenter RL, Neal JM. Epidural anesthesia and analgesia. Their role in postoperative outcome. *Anesthesiology* 1995;82:1474.

16. Wu CL, Fleisher LA. Outcomes research in regional anesthesia and analgesia. *Anesth Analg* 2000;91:1232.

17. Malinovsky JM, Le Normand L, Lepage JY, et al. The urodynamic effects of intravenous opioids and ketoprofen in humans. *Anesth Analg* 1998;87:456-461.

18. Hayek SM, Deer TR. Intrathecal therapy for cancer and non-cancer pain. A systematic review. *Pain Physician* 2011;14:219–248.

Chapter 8

Complementary and Alternative Medicine

Amaresh Vydyanathan, Zachary Leuschner, and Karina Gritsenko

Introduction

Pain is one of the most prevalent conditions for which people seek medical attention. With increasing emphasis on pain therapy in recent years, the use of complementary and alternative medicine (CAM) for the treatment of pain has also gained importance and grown in usage. For example, an estimated 1 million people in the United States use acupuncture yearly, primarily for pain relief (1–3). This increase is thought to be related to the ineffectiveness of conventional therapy for certain pain conditions, increasing recognition of CAM, and improved access to CAM treatment modalities as part of a multidisciplinary model of pain treatment.

Although the use of CAM is gaining wider acceptance, there is still the specter of unproven efficacy with CAM (4). Likewise, in perioperative pain treatment, some individual studies have shown benefits to certain CAM modalities, but other studies do not show any benefit. This chapter provides an evidence-based overview of some of the CAM modalities commonly used in the treatment of chronic and acute pain conditions.

CAM modalities can be broadly divided into the following categories (adapted from the *National Center for Complementary and Alternative Medicine*):

1. Alternative medical systems: acupuncture, homeopathy, reflexology
2. Mind–body medicine: hypnosis, tai chi, biofeedback, guided imagery, relaxation techniques, creative therapy (e.g., music therapy), support groups
3. Manipulative and body-based practices: spinal manipulation, massage therapy, transcutaneous electrical nerve stimulation (TENS)
4. Biologic-based therapy: herbal supplements, nutritional supplements
5. Energy therapies: Reiki, healing touch

Alternative Medical Systems

Acupuncture

Acupuncture, a modality of Chinese traditional medicine, has existed since the first century B.C. and is considered one of the most enduring CAM modalities.

It is based on the concept of *qi*, or life force, which runs through the body and serves to protect the body. When the *qi* is disrupted, the result is disease, or pain. The aim of acupuncture is to rebalance *qi*.

Traditionally, acupuncture is performed using 32-gauge needles, inserted at one or more of over 350 precise points that lie along meridians, and/or points that are painful to palpation. The rebalancing of *qi* is performed by stimulating these needles either manually or electrically with heat (5) (Fig. 8.1).

Research into the mechanism of action of acupuncture has shown reproducible neurobiologic effects, including activation of A-beta fibers and concomitant reduction in pain transmission (6), increased production of endogenous opioid peptides (7), and reduction in hyperalgesic responses through activation of serotonergic pathways (8). Recent functional MRI studies show that acupuncture induced activation over limbic areas and reduced activity over the rostral anterior cingulated cortex (rACC) (9).

Clinically, acupuncture is one of the most extensively studied CAM modalities. In the treatment of postoperative pain the evidence is unclear. While some

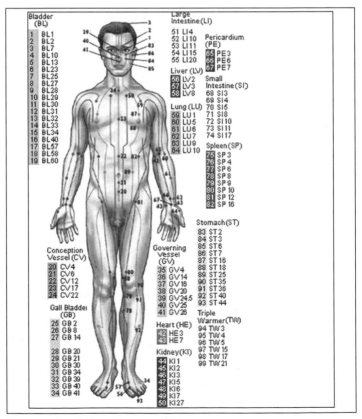

Figure 8.1 Sample Map of Acupuncture Points.

studies and systematic reviews have shown benefit to using acupuncture and acupressure modalities in postoperative pain (10–13), other studies have shown minimal or no benefit (14–18). In chronic pain treatment, systematic reviews and independent studies have shown effectiveness of acupuncture in low back pain (19), headaches (20), temporomandibular joint pain (21), myofascial pain (22), and knee pain (23), while its effect on neck pain (24) and neuropathic pain (25) is unclear.

Homeopathy

Homeopathy is a system of medicine developed in Germany 200 years ago. The two primary principles of the system are the "principle of similars" (diseases are cured by substances that produce similar symptoms in healthy people) and the "principle of dilution" (the lower the dose of medicine given, the greater the effectiveness).

While there is some evidence that homeopathy is efficacious in the treatment of fibromyalgia (26) and rheumatoid arthritis (27), the evidence is meager, and there is no definitive evidence of consistent effectiveness of homeopathy in treating pain.

Mind–Body Medicine

Hypnosis

Hypnosis involves invoking heightened imagination and relaxation in the patient via suggestive techniques. The components of a hypnotic treatment are becoming absorbed in an object of concentration, proceeding to dissociation from the surrounding environment, followed by suggestibility. This enables the patient to experience changes in sensation, thought, and behavior not usually accessible to the conscious mind (28).

Hypnosis has been shown to be of benefit in treating pain in patients with headache, arthritis, cancer, low back pain, and musculoskeletal pain (28–30). Typically there is benefit in adding hypnosis to the treatment strategy (30). Hypnosis has also been proposed as useful in treating acute pain conditions, but there is no good evidence substantiating any benefit to its use in this setting (15,16).

Biofeedback

Biofeedback involves the use of devices to facilitate conscious control of physiologic body functions that are normally controlled unconsciously, including autonomic functions such as heart rate, respiratory rate, muscle tension, and so forth, to promote pain relief and relaxation. During the treatment, the patient is attached to a monitor that records physiologic function and displays it to the patient as an auditory or visual stimulus so that the patient can learn to control the stimulus and in turn control the physiologic response. Examples include electromyographic feedback provided in myofascial pain or thermal feedback provided in migraine.

The mechanisms underlying biofeedback are unknown. The benefit is believed to be from improved control of the dysregulated autonomic system (31) and providing an improved sense of relaxation. While studied most extensively in the treatment of temporomandibular joint pain, it has been found to be effective in treating pain from headache, fibromyalgia, back pain, and irritable bowel syndrome and even acute pain (32, 33). Recently, biofeedback using functional MRI to help patients control activation of the rACC has shown promise (34).

Tai Chi

Tai chi is an ancient Chinese martial art that combines slow, controlled movements with diaphragmatic breathing and meditation. The practice dates to the 13th century, although its health benefits are only now being studied. A 2009 meta-analysis of randomized control trials on the effectiveness of tai chi for chronic musculoskeletal pain showed a significant reduction in scores on pain and disability scales (35). Another study in rheumatoid arthritis patients found improved muscle function and reduction in reported pain (36).

Manipulative and Body-Based Treatments

Spinal Manipulation

Spinal manipulation refers to hands-on treatment based on joint and muscle mobilization in and around the spine. The American Chiropractic Association defines it as a passive manual maneuver "during which the three joint complex is carried beyond the normal physiological range of movement without exceeding the boundaries of anatomic integrity." It is based on the premise that joint restriction contributes to pain and utilizes a low- or high-velocity thrust at the end of passive range of movement in an attempt to increase the joint's range of motion. It has been found to be effective in acute and chronic musculoskeletal pain disorders, including low back pain (37–39).

The mechanism of pain control with spinal manipulation is unknown. Manipulation activates spinal serotonergic and noradrenergic receptors that mediate analgesia (40). It has also been proposed that manipulation increases circulation and increases endorphin levels (41).

Massage Therapy

Massage therapy involves application of pressure and movement by the hands over soft tissues to produce a therapeutic effect. Classic massage by itself has different forms:

1. *Effleurage* involves stroking movements.
2. *Petrissage* involves kneading movements in a centripetal fashion.
3. *Friction massage* involves applying pressure with the ball of the thumb in a circular pattern to loosen scars and adhesions.
4. *Tapotement* involves applying percussive cups in series.

Sports massage involves aggressive massage techniques, mainly in preparation for and subsequent to athletic events. Shiatsu involves the application of pressure over predetermined points along energy lines to improve energy flow.

Massage is theorized to improve circulation and cause breakdown of soft tissue adhesions. It is also thought to reduce pain transmission secondary to

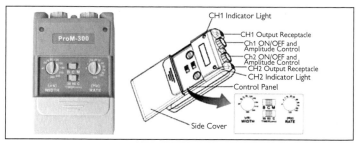

Figure 8.2 Illustration of a TENS Unit.

stimulation of large-diameter nerve fibers. The evidence for the efficacy of massage therapy in treating pain is minimal, with little objective research supporting its use (42–44).

Transcutaneous Electrical Nerve Stimulation and Percutaneous Electrical Nerve Stimulation

Transcutaneous electrical nerve stimulation (TENS) and percutaneous electrical nerve stimulation involve application of electrical stimulation across the skin (Fig. 8.2). They are used in the treatment of persistently painful musculoskeletal conditions such as sciatica, low back and cervical axial pain, and acute postoperative pain (45–47). The theoretical basis of action is related to the gate control theory of pain: pain transmission through C fibers is blocked by stimulation of large A fibers. There is likely a more complex mechanism of action involving the release of endogenous opioids and activation of other neurophysiologic processes involved (48). The advantage of TENS is its customizability, the ability to use it on almost any area of the body, and minimal side effects (48). TENS is contraindicated in patients with demand-mode pacemakers and in pregnancy.

TENS is one of the CAM modalities most extensively studied in postoperative pain states. Multiple studies involving orthopaedic and thoracic surgeries have shown benefit with the use of TENS in terms of postoperative pain levels, with concomitant reduction in opioid use (49–53), and systematic reviews of the literature further strengthen the evidence for its benefit (54, 55).

Biologic-Based Therapy

Herbal Therapy

Herbal therapy involves using plant-derived products to alleviate medical conditions. It has recently gained popularity as patients look to natural treatments for medical conditions. Pertaining to pain treatment, *Tanacetum parthenium* (feverfew) is used to treat migraines, while *Harpagophytum procumbens* (devil's claw) and *Salix alba* (white willow bark) are used commonly to treat low back pain.

A Cochrane review showed a positive effect with the use of feverfew in migraine prophylaxis (56). Parthenolide, an active ingredient in feverfew, has serotonin-inhibiting properties that may contribute to its efficacy in migraine prophylaxis (57). Similarly, studies have shown evidence of the effectiveness of devil's claw and white willow bark in the treatment of low back pain, but the studies have methodological deficiencies and the evidence is meager (58, 59).

There are many other herbal remedies used to treat pain, but the evidentiary support is minimal. Further, herbal remedies may have significant side effects; thus, it is important to elicit a history of herbal medicine use during patient evaluation. Information on herbal supplements is available at the *National Center for Complementary and Alternative Medicine* website (nccam.nih.gov).

Nutritional Supplements

These are nonherbal supplements used to treat a variety of medical conditions, including pain. Some of the most common supplements are glucosamine and chondroitin sulfate for osteoarthritis and other orthopaedic conditions (60), fish oil for inflammatory conditions (61) and pain, and vitamins (i.e., vitamin D) for pain conditions. While these examples have significant anecdotal support for their use, studies of these supplements are few, are often uncontrolled, or have methodological flaws, so their efficacy is unproven. They do not have as many reported side effects as herbal supplements.

Energy Therapy

Energy medicine is a branch of CAM that operates on the belief that the healer can channel healing energy into the patient using various methods. The *National Center for Complementary and Alternative Medicine* distinguishes this branch of CAM based on the source of energy: the use of scientifically observable energy is called veritable energy medicine (e.g., magnet therapy), and the use of undetectable energy is called putative energy medicine (e.g., Reiki).

While there is evidence of the benefit of energy therapy in the treatment of pain conditions (62, 63), the veracity of the findings have been questioned. Nonetheless, energy therapy remains a popular component of CAM treatments used for pain conditions, and more studies researching its efficacy are forthcoming.

Conclusion

CAM approaches to the treatment of pain represent an evolving specialty. While there remain doubts regarding the efficacy of CAM approaches in pain control given the paucity of literature, the growing body of evidence makes these methods an integral part of any multidisciplinary model of pain treatment.

References

1. Eisenberg DM, Davis RB, Ettner SL, et al. Trends in alternative medicine use in the United States, 1990–1997: results of a follow-up national survey. *JAMA* 1998;280:1569–1575.

2. Rao JK, Mihaliak K, Kroenke K, Bradley J, Tierney WM, Weinberger M. Use of complementary therapies for arthritis among patients of rheumatologists. *Ann Intern Med* 1999;131:409–416.

3. Bullock ML, Pheley AM, Kiresuk TJ, Lenz SK, Culliton PD. Characteristics and complaints of patients seeking therapy at a hospital-based alternative medicine clinic. *J Altern Complement Med* 1997;3:31–37.

4. Koretz RL, Rotblatt M. Complementary and alternative medicine in gastroenterology: the good, the bad, and the ugly. *Clin Gastroenterol Hepatol* 2004;2:957–967.

5. Weiner DK, Ernst E. Complementary and alternative approaches to the treatment of persistent musculoskeletal pain. *Clin J Pain* 2004;20:244–255.

6. Lewith GT, Kenyon JN. Physiological and psychological explanations for the mechanism of acupuncture as a treatment for chronic pain. *Soc Sci Med* 1984;19:1367–1378.

7. He LF. Involvement of endogenous opioid peptides in acupuncture analgesia. *Pain* 1987;31:99–121.

8. Yonehara N. Influence of serotonin receptor antagonists on substance P and serotonin release evoked by tooth pulp stimulation with electro-acupuncture in the trigeminal nucleus cudalis of the rabbit. *Neurosci Res* 2001;40:45–51.

9. Wu MT, Sheen JM, Chuang KH, et al. Neuronal specificity of acupuncture response: a fMRI study with electroacupuncture. *NeuroImage* 2002;16:1028–1037.

10. Coura LE, Manoel CH, Poffo R, Bedin A, Westphal GA. Randomised, controlled study of preoperative electroacupuncture for postoperative pain control after cardiac surgery. *Acupuncture Med* 2011;29:16–20.

11. Langenbach MR, Aydemir-Dogruyol K, Issel R, Sauerland S. Randomized sham-controlled trial of acupuncture for postoperative pain control after stapled haemorrhoidopexy. *Colorectal Dis* 2012;14:e486–491.

12. Yeh ML, Chung YC, Chen KM, Tsou MY, Chen HH. Acupoint electrical stimulation reduces acute postoperative pain in surgical patients with patient-controlled analgesia: a randomized controlled study. *Alternative Therapies in Health and Medicine* 2010;16:10–18.

13. Asher GN, Jonas DE, Coeytaux RR, et al. Auriculotherapy for pain management: a systematic review and meta-analysis of randomized controlled trials. *J Altern Complement Med* 2010;16:1097–1108.

14. Holzer A, Leitgeb U, Spacek A, Wenzl R, Herkner H, Kettner S. Auricular acupuncture for postoperative pain after gynecological surgery: a randomized controlled trail. *Minerva Anestesiologica* 2011;77:298–304.

15. Hunt K, Ernst E. The evidence base for complementary medicine in children: a critical overview of systematic reviews. *Arch Dis Child* 2011;96:769–776.

16. Roberts M, Brodribb W, Mitchell G. Reducing the pain: a systematic review of postdischarge analgesia following elective orthopedic surgery. *Pain Med* 2012;13:711–727.

17. Wetzel B, Pavlovic D, Kuse R, et al. The effect of auricular acupuncture on fentanyl requirement during hip arthroplasty: a randomized controlled trial. *Clin J Pain* 2011;27:262–267.

18. Yeh ML, Tsou MY, Lee BY, Chen HH, Chung YC. Effects of auricular acupressure on pain reduction in patient-controlled analgesia after lumbar spine surgery. *Acta Anaesthesiol Taiwanica* 2010;48:80–86.

19. Ernst E, White AR. Acupuncture for back pain: a meta-analysis of randomized controlled trials. *Arch Intern Med* 1998;158:2235–2241.

20. Melchart D, Linde K, Fischer P, et al. Acupuncture for recurrent headaches: a systematic review of randomized controlled trials. *Cephalalgia* 1999;19:779–786; discussion 65.

21. Fink M, Rosted P, Bernateck M, Stiesch-Scholz M, Karst M. Acupuncture in the treatment of painful dysfunction of the temporomandibular joint—a review of the literature. *Forsch Komplementmed* 2006;13:109–115.

22. Lewit K. The needle effect in the relief of myofascial pain. *Pain* 1979;6:83–90.

23. White A, Foster NE, Cummings M, Barlas P. Acupuncture treatment for chronic knee pain: a systematic review. *Rheumatology (Oxford)* 2007;46:384–390.

24. White AR, Ernst E. A systematic review of randomized controlled trials of acupuncture for neck pain. *Rheumatology (Oxford)* 1999;38:143–147.

25. Shlay JC, Chaloner K, Max MB, et al. Acupuncture and amitriptyline for pain due to HIV-related peripheral neuropathy: a randomized controlled trial. Terry Beirn Community Programs for Clinical Research on AIDS. *JAMA* 1998;280:1590–1595.

26. Perry R, Terry R, Ernst E. A systematic review of homoeopathy for the treatment of fibromyalgia. *Clin Rheumatol* 2010;29:457–464.

27. Jonas WB, Linde K, Ramirez G. Homeopathy and rheumatic disease. *Rheum Dis Clin North Am* 2000;26:117–123.

28. Spiegel D, Moore R. Imagery and hypnosis in the treatment of cancer patients. *Oncology (Williston Park)* 1997;11:1179–1195.

29. Patterson DR, Jensen MP. Hypnosis and clinical pain. *Psychol Bull* 2003;129:495–521.

30. Montgomery GH, DuHamel KN, Redd WH. A meta-analysis of hypnotically induced analgesia: how effective is hypnosis? *Int J Clin Exp Hypnosis* 2000;48:138–153.

31. Rainville P, Bao QV, Chretien P. Pain-related emotions modulate experimental pain perception and autonomic responses. *Pain* 2005;118:306–318.

32. Carroll D, Seers K. Relaxation for the relief of chronic pain: a systematic review. *J Adv Nurs* 1998;27:476–487.

33. Seers K, Carroll D. Relaxation techniques for acute pain management: a systematic review. *J Adv Nurs* 1998;27:466–475.

34. deCharms RC, Maeda F, Glover GH, et al. Control over brain activation and pain learned by using real-time functional MRI. *Proc Natl Acad Sci USA* 2005;102:18626–18631.

35. Hall A, Maher C, Latimer J, Ferreira M. The effectiveness of Tai Chi for chronic musculoskeletal pain conditions: a systematic review and meta-analysis. *Arthritis Rheumatism* 2009;61:717–724.

36. Uhlig T, Fongen C, Steen E, Christie A, Odegard S. Exploring Tai Chi in rheumatoid arthritis: a quantitative and qualitative study. *BMC Musculoskeletal Disorders* 2010;11:43.

37. Bronfort G. Spinal manipulation: current state of research and its indications. *Neurol Clin* 1999;17:91–111.

38. van Tulder MW, Koes BW, Bouter LM. Conservative treatment of acute and chronic nonspecific low back pain. A systematic review of randomized controlled trials of the most common interventions. *Spine* 1997;22:2128–2156.

39. Assendelft WJ, Morton SC, Yu EI, Suttorp MJ, Shekelle PG. Spinal manipulative therapy for low back pain. A meta-analysis of effectiveness relative to other therapies. *Ann Intern Med* 2003;138:871–881.

40. Skyba DA, Radhakrishnan R, Rohlwing JJ, Wright A, Sluka KA. Joint manipulation reduces hyperalgesia by activation of monoamine receptors but not opioid or GABA receptors in the spinal cord. *Pain* 2003;106:159–168.

41. Vernon HT, Dhami MS, Howley TP, Annett R. Spinal manipulation and beta-endorphin: a controlled study of the effect of a spinal manipulation on plasma beta-endorphin levels in normal males. *J Manip Physiol Therapeutics* 1986;9:115–123.

42. Imamura M, Furlan AD, Dryden T, Irvin E. Evidence-informed management of chronic low back pain with massage. *Spine J* 2008;8:121–133.

43. Callaghan MJ. The role of massage in the management of the athlete: a review. *Br J Sports Med* 1993;27:28–33.

44. Furlan AD, Imamura M, Dryden T, Irvin E. Massage for low back pain: an updated systematic review within the framework of the Cochrane Back Review Group. *Spine* 2009;34:1669–1684.

45. Ghoname EA, Craig WF, White PF, et al. Percutaneous electrical nerve stimulation for low back pain: a randomized crossover study. *JAMA* 1999;281:818–823.

46. Ghoname EA, White PF, Ahmed HE, Hamza MA, Craig WF, Noe CE. Percutaneous electrical nerve stimulation: an alternative to TENS in the management of sciatica. *Pain* 1999;83:193–199.

47. Ghoname EA, Craig WF, White PF. Use of percutaneous electrical nerve stimulation (PENS) for treating ECT-induced headaches. *Headache* 1999;39:502–505.

48. Sluka KA, Walsh D. Transcutaneous electrical nerve stimulation: basic science mechanisms and clinical effectiveness. *J Pain* 2003;4:109–121.

49. Lan F, Ma YH, Xue JX, Wang TL, Ma DQ. Transcutaneous electrical nerve stimulation on acupoints reduces fentanyl requirement for postoperative pain relief after total hip arthroplasty in elderly patients. *Minerva Anestesiologica* 2012;78:887–895.

50. Fiorelli A, Morgillo F, Milione R, et al. Control of post-thoracotomy pain by transcutaneous electrical nerve stimulation: effect on serum cytokine levels, visual analogue scale, pulmonary function and medication. *Eur J Cardiothoracic Surg* 2012;41:861–868.

51. Kara B, Baskurt F, Acar S, et al. The effect of TENS on pain, function, depression, and analgesic consumption in the early postoperative period with spinal surgery patients. *Turkish Neurosurgery* 2011;21:618–624.

52. Lima PM, Farias RT, Carvalho AC, da Silva PN, Ferraz Filho NA, de Brito RF. Transcutaneous electrical nerve stimulation after coronary artery bypass graft surgery. *Revista Brasileira de Cirurgia Cardiovascular* 2011;26:591–596.

53. Silva MB, de Melo PR, de Oliveira NM, Crema E, Fernandes LF. Analgesic effect of transcutaneous electrical nerve stimulation after laparoscopic cholecystectomy. *Am J Phys Med Rehab* 2012;91:652–657.

54. Sbruzzi G, Silveira SA, Silva DV, Coronel CC, Plentz RD. Transcutaneous electrical nerve stimulation after thoracic surgery: systematic review and meta-analysis of 11 randomized trials. *Revista Brasileira de Cirurgia Cardiovascular* 2012;27:75–87.

55. Bjordal JM, Johnson MI, Ljunggreen AE. Transcutaneous electrical nerve stimulation (TENS) can reduce postoperative analgesic consumption. A meta-analysis with assessment of optimal treatment parameters for postoperative pain. *Eur J Pain* 2003;7:181–188.

56. Pittler MH, Ernst E. Feverfew for preventing migraine. *Cochrane Database Syst Rev*:CD002286, 2004.

57. Heptinstall S, White A, Williamson L, Mitchell JR. Extracts of feverfew inhibit granule secretion in blood platelets and polymorphonuclear leucocytes. *Lancet* 1985;1:1071–1074.

58. Chrubasik S, Eisenberg E, Balan E, Weinberger T, Luzzati R, Conradt C. Treatment of low back pain exacerbations with willow bark extract: a randomized double-blind study. *Am J Med* 2000;109:9–14.

59. Gagnier JJ, van Tulder M, Berman B, Bombardier C. Herbal medicine for low back pain. *Cochrane Database Syst Rev:*CD004504, 2006.

60. McAlindon TE, LaValley MP, Gulin JP, Felson DT. Glucosamine and chondroitin for treatment of osteoarthritis: a systematic quality assessment and meta-analysis. *JAMA* 2000;283:1469–1475.

61. Gil A. Polyunsaturated fatty acids and inflammatory diseases. *Biomedicine & Pharmacotherapy* 2002;56:388–396.

62. Post-White J, Kinney ME, Savik K, Gau JB, Wilcox C, Lerner I. Therapeutic massage and healing touch improve symptoms in cancer. *Integrative Cancer Therapies* 2003;2:332–344.

63. Olson K, Hanson J, Michaud M. A phase II trial of Reiki for the management of pain in advanced cancer patients. *J Pain Symptom Manage* 2003;26:990–997.

Chapter 9

Chronic Pain Patients and Other Coexisting Conditions

Dmitri Souzdalnitski, Joseph Walker III, and
Richard W. Rosenquist

Approximately 230 million major surgical operations are performed worldwide each year (1). It is estimated that up to 35% of adults suffer from chronic pain, and it is likely that a substantial number of patients with preexisting chronic pain present for surgery each year. A major concern for these patients is whether their pain will be controlled following their surgery. This concern is justified, as studies confirm that these patients are more likely to have poor pain control and may experience an exacerbation of their preexisting chronic pain condition in the postoperative period (2).

Perioperative pain control is directly related to clinical outcomes, length of hospital stay, and patient satisfaction. A considerable body of evidence demonstrates the medical, social, and economic benefits of adequate perioperative pain control. Yet to date there are limited perioperative pain control guidelines to address three challenging patient populations: (a) those with chronic pain, (b) those with chronic pain and substance abuse, and (c) those with chronic pain, substance abuse, and a psychiatric diagnosis. In fact, there are no guidelines outlining best practices for postoperative pain control in patients with chronic pain (3). Many factors related to chronic pain, as well as a dearth of publications addressing this group of patients, make it difficult to create perioperative guidelines.

Several structural, functional, psychological, and social markers are linked to chronic pain (4). However, questions remain regarding how different organ systems change and adapt in the patient with chronic pain. Specifically, what pathological changes occur in the neurologic, psychiatric, endocrine, immune, cardiovascular, respiratory, metabolic, and musculoskeletal systems in patients with chronic pain? Recent data from structural, functional, and molecular imaging studies may shed some light on this question and support the notion that chronic pain has characteristics of a distinct disease rather than simply being a constellation of symptoms (Fig. 9.1). In addition to various pathological changes that occur in the neurologic, endocrine, immune, cardiovascular, respiratory, metabolic, and musculoskeletal systems there are psychological and social changes linked to chronic pain. Figure 9.1 is an example of the cyclical untoward biological, social, and psychological events that often result from an untreated chronic pain disorder.

This chapter provides an overview of safe and effective preoperative, intraoperative, and postoperative pain management techniques in patients with chronic pain.

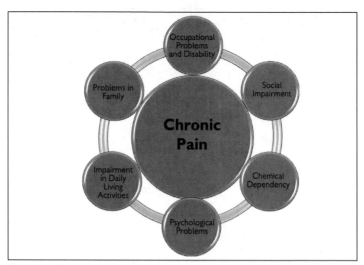

Figure 9.1 Biopsychosocial Issues Resulting from Chronic Pain.

Perioperative Chronic Pain Management in Opioid-Tolerant Patients

Preoperative Period

Optimal perioperative pain management for the patient with chronic pain ideally begins before surgery with an appropriate consultation and evaluation. This starts with a thorough patient history that includes detailed medication use, past surgeries, prior anesthetics, prior procedures, psychiatric history, and any history of substance abuse. In addition, a physical examination should be performed, available images should be reviewed, and any type of implanted pain-management devices should be identified. This should be followed by development of a perioperative pain-control plan that should be discussed in detail with the patient to minimize anxiety and create realistic expectations about what can and will be done to provide adequate perioperative pain control. Without adequate postoperative pain-control strategies, this group of patients may not be able to tolerate early restoration of activity due to low pain thresholds and a high sensitivity to pain. Whenever possible, all anesthesia-related concerns should be answered preoperatively (Table 9.1).

Intraoperative and Postoperative Period

The presence of chronic pain affects the intraoperative anesthetic management, and ongoing use of opioids and antidepressants increases anesthetic requirements during surgery. Changes in intraoperative management may also influence postoperative pain management. Some anesthetic agents may improve postoperative pain management in patients with chronic pain and ongoing opioid use. Propofol has long been considered nonanalgesic; nonetheless, patients anesthetized with propofol appear to experience less pain than those

Table 9.1 Adjuvant Analgesic Medications for Postoperative Management of the Chronic Pain Patient

Antiepileptic Medications

• Continue antiepileptics if the patient takes these medications for chronic pain, neuropathy, or a seizure disorder and if there are no contraindications.

• Consider the use of pregabalin or gabapentin for preemptive analgesia.

• Rapid withdrawal from antiepileptics may trigger seizures, anxiety, and depression.

Nonsteroidal Anti-inflammatory Drugs (NSAIDs) and Acetaminophen

• Continue oral or intravenous NSAIDs or acetaminophen after surgery unless contraindicated or opposed by the surgeon.

Antidepressants and Antipsychotics

• Continue tricyclic antidepressants, selective serotonin reuptake inhibitors (SSRIs), and serotonin–norepinephrine reuptake inhibitors in the perioperative period unless contraindicated.

• Watch for adverse effects of tricyclic antidepressants (sedation, delirium, or other anticholinergic effects, particularly in elderly patients).

• Continue antipsychotics; monitor for signs of neuroleptic malignant syndrome in the acute postoperative setting (hyperthermia, hypertonicity of skeletal muscles, fluctuating levels of consciousness, and autonomic nervous system instability).

• Avoid meperidine combination with SSRIs (paroxetine, fluoxetine, sertraline, citalopram, and others), and monoamine oxidase inhibitor antidepressants (phenelzine, selegiline, tranylcypromine, and others), as these combinations may produce "serotonin syndrome."

Axiolytics

• Antianxiety medications should be continued prior to and after surgery.

• When considering clonidine or dexmedetomidine, continue the preadmission dose of benzodiazepines in the postoperative period to avoid withdrawal symptoms.

• Watch for excessive sedation, potentiated by an escalation in the opioid dose.

Other Adjunctive Medications

• Alpha-2-receptor agonists (dexmedetomidine, clonidine)

• N-methyl-D-aspartate (NMDA) receptor antagonists (ketamine, methadone, potentially nitrous oxide and magnesium)

• Cholinergic receptor agonists (nicotine, neostigmine)

• Corticosteroids

Other Adjunctive Strategies

• Identification of dose, type of opioid (and other pain management medications), history of substance abuse, quality of previous anesthesia

• Education of patient and surgical team on postoperative chronic pain management and preemptive analgesia (premedication, preemptive local anesthetic infiltration, preemptive epidural), multimodal postoperative chronic pain management

• Complement the preoperative discussion with multimedia information.

• Pre-rehabilitation: augmenting functional capacity before surgery

• Early rehabilitation

• Effective use of regional anesthesia and analgesia

anesthetized with sevoflurane (5). This intraoperative finding may also apply to patients with chronic pain. Intraoperative administration of a variety of medications with N-methyl-D-aspartic acid (NMDA) receptor antagonist properties such as ketamine (6), magnesium (7), and methadone (8) has also been shown to reduce postoperative opioid requirements in surgical patients. One meta-analysis demonstrated that total intravenous (IV) anesthesia produced better patient satisfaction in ambulatory settings than inhalational general anesthesia (9). Nitrous oxide is also an effective inhibitor of NMDA receptors, even in subanesthetic concentrations.

Clinical Estimation of Opioid Dosing

Despite weak evidence for improvements in quality of life or function, the number of patients with chronic pain treated with opioids has increased dramatically over the past decade (10). In these opioid-tolerant patients, large doses of opioids are often necessary to control postoperative pain (11). The perioperative management of patients with acute-on-chronic surgical pain and opioid tolerance often requires escalation of opioid doses by a factor of two to four. This is due to a downregulation of opioid receptors in opioid-dependent patients (11). While the medical, social, and economic advantages of adequate perioperative pain control have been proven, it is important to be aware of the risks associated with opioid dose escalation, particularly respiratory depression and excessive sedation (12). In this clinical situation, multimodal pain management strategies employing non-opioid analgesics may be more effective than opioid monotherapy.

Preoperative Opioid Dosing

On the morning of surgery, the routine morning dose of opioids should be taken. If a transdermal opioid delivery system is in use, it should be maintained. If patients do not take their morning opioid dose, they will need to be treated with an equivalent loading dose of opioids preoperatively (12). This can be accomplished either by using an oral medication such as morphine oral elixir (up to 2 hours prior to the surgery) or by IV opioids during induction of anesthesia. The perioperative opioid dose can be estimated by a standardized conversion formula (13).

Preoperative Opioid Challenge and Other Tests

Estimating an effective dose for opioid analgesia in the opioid-dependent patient remains a difficult task. Opioid-dependent patients may paradoxically experience severe postoperative pain but also be at the edge of opioid overdose due to their increased opioid requirements. A variety of nociceptive stimulation methods, including heat injury, pressure algometry, and electrical stimulation, can be useful in predicting the intensity of postoperative pain in opioid-dependent patients (14).

Opioid Conversion and Rotation

While it is recommended to continue the same dose and type of opioids, including the morning of surgery, the need for conversion and rotation of opioids during the perioperative period is almost inevitable (11). There are differing opinions regarding the conversion of oral to IV opioids and regarding opioid rotation (15). In most situations, IV or intramuscular (IM) doses of opioids are less than oral doses. This is because parenteral administration bypasses both gastrointestinal absorption and first-pass hepatic clearance/metabolism. For example, IV morphine has a bioavailability and systemic potency three times greater than equipotent oral doses. Oxycodone is an exception, and extended-release oral oxycodone has a bioavailability that is more than 80% of an equivalent IV dose. The baseline oral dose of oxycodone can be approximated by similar doses of IV morphine (1–1.5 mg oral oxycodone = 1 mg IV morphine) (11). Ideally, patient-specific variables need to be taken into consideration when converting between routes and dosages of opioid medications using conversion tables. These variables, including age, sex, and past medical history, may change the metabolism and excretion of opioids and as a result the appropriate dose of medication (15, 16).

Opioid rotation involves changing one opioid to another in an effort to improve therapeutic response or reduce side effects (15). The specific mechanisms by which opioid rotation improves the overall response to therapy are not completely understood but may be related to incomplete cross-tolerance. It is well established that different opioid medications act on different types or subtypes of opioid receptors. Opioid rotation may lead to a decrease in tolerance, total dose, and toxicity by simply having a different opioid act on a different opioid receptor. For example, in addition to acting on opiate receptors, methadone is also an NMDA receptor antagonist. Methadone may exert its effects by acting on two distinct receptors. Therefore, this medication may be a better choice for certain opioid-dependent patients. In one study, a single bolus of methadone (0.2 mg/kg) before surgical incision was compared with a continuous sufentanil infusion of 0.25 mcg/kg/h after a bolus load of 0.75 mcg/kg of sufentanil in patients undergoing surgery. It was found that methadone reduced postoperative pain by approximately 50% at 48 hours compared to sufentanil. Methadone also reduced the postoperative opioid requirement in patients using IV patient-controlled analgesia (IV-PCA) after the surgery (8).

Postoperative Opioid Dosing

After leaving the operating room, early initiation of IV-PCA lowers the chances of undertreatment. This is accomplished by establishing a basal IV-PCA opioid infusion based on the patient's preoperative baseline opioid dose requirement. This calculated basal rate may be supplemented with additional PCA boluses. Usually a higher-than-normal bolus dose is required to compensate for the patient's opioid tolerance. It is not unusual for the total IV-PCA opioid dose to be two to four times higher than the baseline dose (12). Nevertheless, much lower initial doses may be effective in combination with an opioid rotation strategy.

Basal IV-PCA infusions have proven to be helpful in improving patient analgesia postoperatively. Some practitioners prefer to avoid basal infusions via PCA because of safety concerns; however, this practice may result in severe postoperative pain when intraoperative anesthesia and analgesia start to wear off, and it is reasonable to use basal infusions in opioid-tolerant patients. IV-PCA settings should be evaluated frequently during the first 24 to 48 hours after the surgery. The frequency of evaluation depends on the type of opioid used and the patient's respons e to the therapy. The ratio of patient demand to actual delivery of medication should not exceed 2 to 1 to avoid undertreatment of postoperative pain; ideally, the ratio of the two should match. IV-PCA should be continued until an acceptable level of postoperative pain is achieved. Once an acceptable level of pain is found, the patient can be converted from PCA to oral opioid analgesics. Exceptions can be made if the patient cannot take oral medications.

The PCA setup should allow for the titration of the opioid medications in small increments until an adequate opioid dose is established. Some authors suggest continuing opioid analgesia, at doses of at least half of the preadmission maintenance dose, even in the case of successful neuraxial anesthesia to prevent withdrawal from opioids (11, 12).

Patient Monitoring

Respiratory depression and excessive sedation are real risks, even in opioid-dependent patients. When high doses of opioids are used as the primary form of analgesia, close monitoring of these postsurgical patients should be implemented. The use of pulse oximetry is insufficient as a sole means of monitoring, especially in patients receiving supplemental oxygen. Monitoring must include both respiratory rate and level of sedation. Even judicious dosages of sedatives or anxiolytics in the presence of opioids may significantly increase the risk of respiratory depression.

Perioperative Chronic Pain Management in Special Categories of Patients

History of Substance Abuse

Managing postoperative pain in patients who have a history of substance abuse is clinically challenging. To maximize the potential to deliver adequate perioperative care, it is critical to identify the patient who may be a substance abuser and identify the type of drug currently or previously used, including the dose if possible. There are many clinical clues that can point toward potential substance abuse and many clinical tools that can highlight substance abuse traits (Table 9.2).

The patient who desires opioid medication (i.e., "drug seeking") should not automatically be labeled as a "drug abuser." This mislabeling can lead to miscommunication, improper documentation, poor perioperative pain control, and ultimately a poor perioperative experience. Correct identification of the patient and correct classification of the patient's presenting behavior aid in clinical management (Table 9.3).

It is critical that detoxification is not attempted in the immediate perioperative period. Maintaining the baseline level of opioids is important for achieving adequate perioperative pain control and improving overall patient satisfaction. For patients who are participating in an outpatient methadone substance-abuse treatment program, the IV baseline maintenance dose of methadone is half the oral methadone dose. The exact methadone dose should be verified with the prescribing pharmacy for patient safety reasons.

Some recovering opioid abusers are maintained on buprenorphine. For patients who are participating in outpatient buprenorphine substance-abuse programs, the IV baseline maintenance dose of buprenorphine is routinely equal to the oral buprenorphine dose. Generally, however, the quality of analgesia provided by buprenorphine alone is inadequate. Most often, supplementation with methadone and morphine in addition to buprenorphine should be considered (11). Combined formulations of opioids and opioid antagonists, including

Table 9.2 Perioperative Management of Pain in the Patient with a History of Opioid or Other Substance Abuse

- Identification of patient with history of substance abuse
  - Discuss privacy, confidentiality, and autonomy.
  - Pay attention to the patient's general appearance and manner of communication.
  - Check for relevant notes in the medical records, including history of substance abuse, abnormal laboratory drug screen, repeated early refills, rapid escalation of opioid dose out of proportion to change in clinical picture, multiple telephone encounters with requests to increase the dose of opioids, prescription problems (lost or stolen medications or prescriptions, etc.), multiple emergency-room visits for pain-related issues.
  - Check for state or federal, if available, opioid prescription reports, demonstrating multiple sourcing.
  - Physical exam data (numerous needle marks, skin abscesses, poor peripheral vein access, or disseminated superficial vein thrombosis)
  - Repeat laboratory drug screen, pain medications panel.
  - Inform patient that addiction history will not prevent adequate postoperative pain management.
- Differentiate various types of conditions associated with substance use disorder.
  - "Drug-seeking" patients should not automatically be assumed be "drug abusers."
  - Differentiate "addiction" and "pseudo-addiction," "opioid tolerance" and "pseudo-opioid tolerance," "opioid-induced hyperalgesia," "physical dependence" and "psychological dependence," and other conditions associated with substance use disorder.
  - "Drug seeking" and other related terms can be applied only when the patient's pain is adequately controlled.
- Maintain baseline opioid dose.
  - Do not attempt detoxification for any patient, whether abusing opioids or taking prescribed opioids.
  - Make sure to uphold the baseline level of opioids.
  - Keep in mind that patients may underreport or overreport opioid doses.
- Management of patients participating in substance abuse maintenance programs
  - Verify participation in these programs, and the methadone or buprenorphine doses, for patient safety reasons.
  - The IV baseline maintenance dose of methadone is typically half the oral methadone dose taken by patients who are participating in these programs.
  - Recovering opioid abusers maintained on buprenorphine may continue on this medication in the IV form for postoperative pain control (unless the quality of analgesia provided by buprenorphine is inadequate; supplementation with methadone and morphine may be considered).
- Management of patients treated with combined agonist–antagonist agents preoperatively
  - Combined formulations of opioids and opioid antagonists, including naloxone and naltrexone, should not be used for opioid-dependent patients, because postoperative administration may produce withdrawal symptoms.
  - Naltrexone, a long-acting oral opioid antagonist sometimes used in recovering opioid abusers, should be discontinued at least 24 hours prior to surgery.
- Use of mixed opioid agonist–antagonist drugs postoperatively
  - Inform the surgical team that mixed agonist–antagonist opioids should not be used for substance abusers or opioid-dependent patients (nalbuphine, butorphanol,

(Continued)

Table 9.2 **Continued**

pentazocine, tramadol, and others).

- Consider multimodal regimens, but watch for comorbidities.
  - Multimodal approaches may be useful to spare opioids.
  - Consider multiple comorbidities and commonly accompanying substance abuse states, including viral or ethanol-related liver disease, HIV, lung disease (smoking is common in this patient population), encephalopathy, psychiatric comorbidities, and others.
- Abuse of other substances
  - Substances other than opioids may complicate postoperative chronic pain management.
  - Watch for ethanol abuse and withdrawal.
  - Nicotine patches should be invariably applied to smokers to prevent withdrawal; this may improve their perception of recovery after the surgery.
- Management of substance use at the time of discharge
  - Healthcare providers should address substance abuse issues in a conventional way when the patient is stable and the pain is tolerable.
  - Standard pathways and recovery options should be offered to patients with a history of substance abuse, including alcohol and nicotine.
  - Smokers should be informed about the tight association between chronic nicotine use and chronic back pain.
  - The primary care provider, the addiction treatment maintenance program, and/or the prescribing physician of any opioids and benzodiazepines should be informed about medications given to the patient during hospitalization (because they may show up on routine urine drug screening) as well as the doses of these medications to provide effective continuous care.

Adapted from Souzdalnitski D, Cheng J. Postoperative chronic pain management. In Farag E, ed. *Anesthesia for Spine Surgery*, 1st ed. Cambridge University Press, 2012:312-347.

naloxone and naltrexone, should not be used for opioid-dependent patients because postoperative administration may produce withdrawal symptoms. Naltrexone, a long-acting oral opioid antagonist (sometimes used in recovering opioid abusers), should also be discontinued at least 24 hours prior to surgery (11). Mixed agonist–antagonist opioids should not be used either for substance abusers or for opioid-dependent patients. Since the receptor-binding affinity of buprenorphine or its combination with naloxone ("Suboxone") can be observed for up to 5 days (17), we suggest switching patients who take these medications to regular opioids at least 5 days prior to surgery. The proactive use of non-opioid analgesics, adjuncts, local and regional techniques, and their combinations is also advisable (17).

Substances other than opioids, such as ethyl alcohol and cigarettes, may also complicate postoperative chronic pain management. There is a risk of delirium tremens 3 to 4 days after the last drink, and it may be reasonable to allow the consumption of drinks containing ethyl alcohol in small amounts to avoid this complication. Alternatively, other compounds such as benzodiazepines, clonidine, or others may be helpful in preventing abstinence symptoms. Nicotine patches should be considered for tobacco users to prevent withdrawal. The substance abuse disorder should be addressed in the conventional manner after the patient is stable and the pain is manageable.

Table 9.3 Conditions Associated with Substance Use Disorder and Chronic Opioid Use

- Dependence
  - *Psychological dependence*: need for a specific psychoactive substance either for its positive effects or to avoid negative psychological or physical effects associated with its withdrawal
  - *Physical dependence*: a physiologic state of adaptation to a specific psychoactive substance characterized by the emergence of a withdrawal syndrome during abstinence, which may be relieved totally or in part by readministration of the substance
- Drug-seeking behavior
  - Patient requests additional opioid or other psychoactive medications supply.
  - "Drug seeking" and other related terms can be applied only when the patient's pain is controlled, as it may be an appropriate response to inadequately treated pain.
- Opioid tolerance and pseudo opioid tolerance
  - Opioid tolerance: habituation or desensitization of anti-nociceptive pathways mediated by opioid medications producing a decline in the analgesic effect of normally efficacious doses of opioids
  - *Pseudo-opioid tolerance*: patient may exhibit drug-seeking behavior despite adequate pain relief to prevent reduction in current or future opioid analgesic dose
- Opioid-induced hyperalgesia
  - *Opioid-induced hyperalgesia*: a decline in the analgesic effect of normally efficacious doses of opioids; also defined as a state of nociceptive sensitization caused by exposure to opioids; a paradoxical response to opioids that decreases the overall pain tolerance, probably a result of neuroplastic changes in the peripheral and central nervous systems that lead to sensitization of pro-nociceptive pathways
- Addiction and pseudoaddiction
  - *Addiction*: a pattern of maladaptive behaviors, including loss of control over use, craving and preoccupation with substance use, and continued use despite harm resulting from use (this term is being replaced by the term "substance use disorder with psychological and physical dependence")
  - *Pseudo-addiction*: addiction-like behavior caused by inadequate pain control
- Substance use disorder
  - *Substance dependence disorder* or *substance abuse disorder with psychological or/and physical dependence*
  - *Substance-induced disorders* (intoxication, withdrawal, delirium, psychotic disorders, and others)

Depression, Anxiety, and Other Psychiatric Conditions

Patients with chronic pain are at a higher risk for depression and anxiety than the general population. While a connection between perioperative chronic pain management and clinical problems related to depression and anxiety is recognized, how best to manage this association is still being explored. Literature suggests that clinicians need to be more sensitive to the psychological concerns of patients with depression and/or anxiety undergoing surgery (18, 19). If there are questions about how best to manage a patient's experience during the perioperative period, a brief psychological screening with and/or without a comprehensive assessment from a mental health professional should be immediately considered. Some antidepressant medications have analgesic effects and may contribute to the overall effects of postoperative pain management. Several tricyclic antidepressants, such as duloxetine and milnacipran, are approved for the treatment of chronic neuropathic or myofascial pain. Selective serotonin reuptake inhibitors, tricyclic antidepressants, and serotonin–norepinephrine reuptake inhibitors should be routinely continued in the preoperative dosages because such antidepressants are important elements in the treatment of depression. Adverse effects of tricyclic antidepressants are common, and patients taking them should be reevaluated if there is evidence of sedation and delirium or other anticholinergic effects, particularly in elderly patients. Meperidine should be avoided in combination with selective serotonin reuptake inhibitors (paroxetine, fluoxetine, sertraline, citalopram, and others) and monoamine oxidase inhibitors (phenelzine, selegiline, tranylcypromine, and others). These combinations may produce significant clinical derangements, including hyperreflexia, myoclonus, ataxia, fever, shivering, diaphoresis, diarrhea, anxiety, salivation, and confusion (often termed "serotonin syndrome").

Less than 1% of all patients treated with antipsychotic drugs may develop a neuroleptic malignant syndrome. This is demonstrated as hyperthermia, hypertonicity of the skeletal muscles, fluctuating levels of consciousness, and autonomic nervous system instability. Patients taking antipsychotics should be closely observed in the perioperative period.

References

1. World Health Organization (WHO). *Report on Emergency and Surgical Care.* Available at: http://www.who.int/surgery/en/index.html (Accessed May 15, 2012.)

2. Pizzi LT, Toner R, Foley K, et al. Relationship between potential opioid-related adverse effects and hospital length of stay in patients receiving opioids after orthopedic surgery. *Pharmacotherapy* 2012;32(6):502–514.

3. American Society of Anesthesiologists Task Force on Chronic Pain Management, American Society of Regional Anesthesia and Pain Medicine. Practice guidelines for chronic pain management: an updated report by the American Society of Anesthesiologists Task Force on Chronic Pain Management and the American Society of Regional Anesthesia and Pain Medicine. *Anesthesiology* 2010;112(4):810–833.

4. Tracey I, Bushnell MC. How neuroimaging studies have challenged us to rethink: is chronic pain a disease? *J Pain* 2009;10(11):1113–1120.

5. Tan T, Bhinder R, Carey M, Briggs L. Day-surgery patients anesthetized with propofol have less postoperative pain than those anesthetized with sevoflurane. *Anesth Analg* 2010;111(1):83–85.

6. Yamauchi M, Asano M, Watanabe M, Iwasaki S, Furuse S, Namiki A. Continuous low-dose ketamine improves the analgesic effects of fentanyl patient-controlled analgesia after cervical spine surgery. *Anesth Analg* 2008;107(3):1041–1044.

7. Oguzhan N, Gunday I, Turan A. Effect of magnesium sulfate infusion on sevoflurane consumption, hemodynamics, and perioperative opioid consumption in lumbar disc surgery. *J Opioid Manag* 2008;4(2):105–110.

8. Gottschalk A, Durieux ME, Nemergut EC. Intraoperative methadone improves postoperative pain control in patients undergoing complex spine surgery. *Anesth Analg* 2011;112(1):218–223.

9. Leonova M, Souzdalnitski D. Patient satisfaction is higher with TIVA than with inhalational anesthesia for ambulatory surgery. Available at: http://www.asaabstracts.com (Accessed May 15, 2012).

10. Noble M, Treadwell JR, Tregear SJ, et al. Long-term opioid management for chronic noncancer pain. *Cochrane Database Syst Rev* 2010;(1)(1):CD006605.

11. Mitra S, Sinatra RS. Perioperative management of acute pain in the opioid-dependent patient. *Anesthesiology* 2004;101(1):212–227.

12. Kopf A, Banzhaf A, Stein C. Perioperative management of the chronic pain patient. *Best Pract Res Clin Anaesthesiol* 2005;19(1):59–76.

13. Davis JJ, Swenson JD, Hall RH, et al. Preoperative "fentanyl challenge" as a tool to estimate postoperative opioid dosing in chronic opioid-consuming patients. *Anesth Analg* 2005;101(2):389–395.

14. Werner MU, Mjobo HN, Nielsen PR, Rudin A. Prediction of postoperative pain: a systematic review of predictive experimental pain studies. *Anesthesiology* 2010;112(6):1494–1502.

15. Knotkova H, Fine PG, Portenoy RK. Opioid rotation: the science and the limitations of the equianalgesic dose table. *J Pain Symptom Manage* 2009;38(3):426–439.

16. Stamer UM, Zhang L, Stuber F. Personalized therapy in pain management: where do we stand? *Pharmacogenomics* 2010;11(6):843–864.

17. Gevirtz C, Frost EA, Bryson EO. Perioperative implications of buprenorphine maintenance treatment for opioid addiction. *Int Anesthesiol Clin* 2011;49(1):147–155.

18. Carr EC, Nicky Thomas V, Wilson-Barnet J. Patient experiences of anxiety, depression and acute pain after surgery: a longitudinal perspective. *Int J Nurs Stud* 2005;42(5):521–530.

19. Khan RS, Ahmed K, Blakeway E, et al. Catastrophizing: a predictive factor for postoperative pain. *Am J Surg* 2011;201(1):122–131.

Chapter 10

Special Populations: Pediatric and Elderly Patients

Veronica Carullo, Wilson Almonte, Christine Milner, and Karina Gritsenko

Introduction

The management of pain in the pediatric and elderly populations can be complicated by factors such as age, individual physiology, disease-related changes in physiology, and disease-drug and drug-drug interactions (1, 2). These populations differ from the general adult populations in terms of physiology, pharmacodynamics, pharmacokinetics, perception of pain, and communicability of pain. In the past 25 years, pediatric studies have elucidated that neonates, infants, and children can receive analgesia and anesthesia safely, with appropriate age-related modifications in clinical practice and dosing (2). The pharmacologic management of pain in elderly patients is complicated by the lack of clinical investigations conducted in these patients, particularly frail and cognitively impaired older patients (3).

Perioperative Pain Management in Pediatric Populations

Children suffer from postoperative pain at least to the same extent as their adult counterparts, yet they often receive less analgesia (4, 5). It is now well documented that neonates are born with the ability to perceive pain, as they have considerable maturation of the peripheral, spinal, and supraspinal afferent pain transmission neural pathways by 26 weeks of gestation. Furthermore, the descending inhibitory pathway develops after birth, heightening their sensitivity to noxious stimuli. Neonates' ability to process noxious stimuli has been demonstrated by their response to tissue injury with specific behavior and autonomic, hormonal, and metabolic signs of stress and distress (2, 6, 7). Studies in neonates have shown that pain, if left untreated, can lead to amplified physiologic or behavioral responses to future noxious events as well as the development of chronic pain syndromes (8, 9).

Assessment of Pain in Pediatric Patients

The appropriate assessment of pain in children is the first step in developing an effective pain management plan. Whenever possible, using a self-report method remains the gold standard for determining pain intensity. The Faces Pain Scale is commonly and successfully used in children as young as 3 years of age. Older children, usually above the age of 7 years, can use tools such as the Visual Analog Scale (VAS) or the Numeric Rating Scale (NRS)(10, 11). Neonates, infants, and children under the age of 3 or those unable to communicate are primarily assessed for pain via behavioral or observational pain assessment tools using the child's facial expressions, limb and trunk motor responses, verbal responses, or combinations of behavioral, physiologic, and autonomic measures. Some examples include the Neonatal Infant Pain Scale (NIPS), the Premature Infant Pain Profile (PIPP), the Neonatal Pain, Agitation & Sedation Score (N-PASS), and the Face, Legs, Activity, Cry, Consolability (FLACC) Scale.

Analgesic Pharmacodynamic and Pharmacokinetic Considerations in Children

The physiologic development of children affects the pharmacokinetics of some agents. The liver and kidneys are the most important organs responsible for drug metabolism and clearance. Glomerular filtration rate is diminished in the first week of life, resulting in decreased drug clearance. Although neonates are born with most of the hepatic enzymes intact, there is delayed maturation of the enzyme systems involved in drug conjugation. This affects a neonate's ability to conjugate most analgesics, including opioids and local anesthetics. Furthermore, drug dose requirements vary with age because volume of distribution, half-life, and clearance change during development (12).

Pediatric Pharmacologic Management

Non-Opioids

Acetaminophen is the most widely used analgesic in the pediatric population. It differs from nonsteroidal anti-inflammatory agents (NSAIDs) as it inhibits central cyclooxygenase (COX) as opposed to peripheral COX and has an improved side-effect profile (6). Acetaminophen can be administered orally, rectally, and intravenously. Adults, adolescents, and children demonstrate similar acetaminophen pharmacokinetic disposition, while infants and neonates show reduced clearance and higher exposure (13). Regardless of the route of delivery, the terminal elimination half-life of acetaminophen is approximately 2 to 4 hours and is slightly longer in infants and neonates (14).

NSAIDs provide anti-inflammatory effects via inhibition of COX, thus inhibiting prostaglandin and thromboxane formation. These drugs can be used in combination with opioids, thus reducing opioid dose and related side effects (15). Pharmacokinetic studies of NSAIDs have shown that weight-normalized clearance and volumes of distribution are greater in children than adults, but their elimination half-lives are similar (1). Limited data exist regarding the safety and efficacy of NSAIDs in neonates and young infants. Ketorolac, a peripheral nonselective COX inhibitor, is available in an injectable form and is indicated for use in pediatric patients aged 6 months and older for mild to moderate pain.

The main adverse effects of NSAIDs include nephropathy, gastropathy, and platelet dysfunction. In children, short-term use of NSAIDs is well tolerated, with a low incidence of side effects. There is an increased risk of renal and hepatic toxicity with hypovolemia and cardiac failure, and a significant risk of gastrointestinal bleeding with prolonged use, albeit a significantly lower risk than in adults (12). A quantitative review by Møiniche and colleagues looked at NSAIDs and the risk of operative-site bleeding after tonsillectomy from 25 studies with data from 970 patients and concluded that NSAIDs were associated with a significant increase in reoperation due to bleeding, although they did not have a significant impact on intraoperative blood loss, postoperative bleeding, or hospital readmission rates (16).

Opioids

Opioids are frequently used in the perioperative period for the treatment of moderate to severe pain in children. The weight-normalized clearance of several opioids is diminished in neonates and reaches mature values over the first 2 to 6 months of life (1). The immature hepatic enzyme systems of preterm and term neonates result in decreased conjugation of opioids. In addition, glomerular filtration is reduced in the first week of life, leading to slower elimination of opioid metabolites (12).

Neonates and infants also have an immature ventilatory response to hypoxia, making them vulnerable to airway obstruction, hypercapnia, and hypoxemia (1, 17). The respiratory frequency fails to increase during hypoxia in infants, whereas tidal volume exhibits a biphasic response similar to that in adults (17). Neonates and infants with chronic lung disease have impaired ventilatory reflexes, which may increase their risk of opioid-induced respiratory depression. Neonates not undergoing intubation have a higher frequency of opioid-induced respiratory depression compared to infants over 6 months of age and older children. Thus, neonates receiving opioids should be monitored by continuous pulse oximetry (1).

Please refer to Table 10.1 for dosing of non-opioid and opioid analgesics.

Patient-Controlled Analgesia in Children

Intravenous patient-controlled analgesia (PCA) may be used safely for postoperative pain relief in children if they have the cognitive ability to understand and appropriately use it. Studies have looked at its use in patients as young as 3 years of age (12). The addition of a basal infusion is usually reserved for opioid-tolerant patients or patients who have undergone major operations such as thoracotomies or spinal fusions. Nurse-controlled analgesia is an alternative approach for relieving episodic pain in infants and children. This allows nurses to administer precalculated doses of analgesia after a thorough pain assessment is completed (1, 13). This is considered safe and effective and may eliminate time delays in administration, causing delays in pain relief (13).

Neuraxial Analgesia

The most popular and useful neuraxial block used in pediatric patients in the perioperative period is the single-shot caudal block. This reliable, safe block is appropriate for surgical procedures below the level of the umbilicus. Early studies have determined that the dermatome level of analgesia achieved with single-shot caudal blocks correlates with the volume of local anesthetic injected (18). To attain a

Table 10.1 Pediatric Dosing of Common Intravenous and Oral Analgesics: Recommended Starting Dosages

Medication	PO	IV	Comments
Acetaminophen	10–15 mg/kg/dose Q 4–6 hours, not to exceed 5 doses/day, Max single dose 1 g Max daily dose 90 mg/kg/day or 4 g Preterm neonates – 40 mg/kg/day Term neonates & infants – 60 mg/kg/day	15 mg/kg/dose Q 6 hours, or 12.5 mg/kg Q 4 hours Max single dose 1 g Max daily dose 75 mg/kg/day or 4 g	IV formulation approved November 2010 by FDA for use in children >2 years
Ibuprofen	6–10 mg/kg/dose Q 6 hours Max single dose 600 mg	N/A	
Ketorolac	For children >50 kg: 10 mg PO Q 4–6 hours	0.5mg/kg/dose Q 6 hours Max single dose 30mg; recommended for 1–16 years of age	Recommended duration of therapy not to exceed 5 days
Naproxen	6–10 mg/kg/dose Q 8–12 hours Max single dose 375 mg/dose	N/A	Max daily dose: 24 mg/kg/day or 1100 mg/day
Morphine	0.15–0.3 mg/kg/dose Q 4 hours	0.05–0.1 mg/kg/dose Q 3 hours	Common first line unless patient has renal insufficiency
Hydromorphone	0.03–0.08 mg/kg/dose q4 hours	0.005–0.015 mg/kg/dose	
Oxycodone	0.1–0.2 mg/kg/dose Q4 hours	N/A	
Hydrocodone	0.1–0.15 mg/kg Q4 hours	N/A	
Fentanyl	N/A	1–3 mcg/kg/dose Q 1 hour	Tachyphylaxis and tolerance develops rapidly in children particularly when administered as continuous infusion
Methadone	0.1–0.2 mg/kg Q 4–8 hours	0.05–0.1 mg/kg Q 4–8 hours	Must be titrated carefully to avoid delayed sedation and respiratory depression

sacral or T10 dermatome level, a volume of 0.5 mL/kg is used. For a lower- or mid-thoracic dermatome level, a volume of 1 and 1.25 mL/kg is used, respectively.

Epidural analgesia has been shown to be effective in neonates and infants (1). Epidural catheters used to provide continuous epidural analgesia for pain relief for surgical procedures below the fourth dermatome can be placed at caudal, lumbar, and thoracic sites (6, 13). In neonates, and children up to the age of 6 months, the vertebral column remains largely cartilaginous, allowing for epidural catheter visualization with ultrasound along the length of insertion to confirm placement and rule out catheter migration. The use of ultrasound for this purpose is still under investigation (19). Special attention should be paid to the following when placing direct lumbar or thoracic epidural catheters in children: (a) There is a much shorter distance from the skin to the epidural space, (b) the ligamentum flavum is softer in children, and (c) saline should be used for the loss-of-resistance technique rather than air to avoid a venous air embolus, cord compression, or a patchy block (6).

In children less than 8 years of age, a clinically significant decrease in blood pressure secondary to sympathectomy from central neuraxial blocks is rare, so volume loading prior to blocks is unnecessary. In older children and adolescents, fluids or vasopressors are also rarely required to treat the hemodynamic effects of central neuraxial blocks (20). A serious but rare complication is the development of local anesthetic toxicity from systemic absorption, and caution is needed in patients with reduced capacity for local anesthetic metabolism and excretion.

Several epidural additives have been investigated, including ketamine, opioids, and clonidine. Concerns related to the direct neurotoxic and apoptotic effects of ketamine have recently removed this drug as a useful adjunct to epidural analgesia. Commonly used opioids in pediatric epidurals include fentanyl, hydromorphone, morphine, and sufentanil. At present clonidine is not commercially marketed for pediatric epidural analgesia, but there are many papers investigating its use in single-shot analgesia and as an adjuvant to local anesthetics in epidural infusions, particularly in neonates (20). The epidural and caudal dose is 1 to 2 micrograms/kg followed by an infusion of 0.05 to 0.33 micrograms/kg/hour. When used as an adjunct to epidural anesthesia, clonidine can augment and prolong the duration of analgesia (6).

In children, spinal anesthesia generally is used for procedures that are 60 to 75 minutes or less in duration (20). The advantages of this mode of anesthesia include rapid return to the child's baseline alertness, normal appetite, and decreased analgesic and anesthetic side effects (20). In neonates, spinal anesthesia can be used as the sole intraoperative anesthetic for inguinal hernia repair (19).

Spinal anesthesia reduces the risk of postoperative apnea, especially in those infants who are at greatest risk following general anesthesia: infants born at less than 37 weeks gestational age, infants less than 60 weeks postconceptional age at the time of surgery, or infants with continuing apnea of prematurity (21).

Regional Techniques

The consensus of pediatric anesthesiologists is that regional blocks can be performed safely in anesthetized children (6, 21). The incidence of complications with the use of regional techniques in children is comparable to that in adults (21). Specific peripheral block techniques are beyond the scope of this chapter.

Table 10.2 Pediatric Local Anesthetic Dosing: Maximum Dosage		
Medication	Epidural/Peripheral Single Shot	Epidural Continuous Infusion
Lidocaine	5 mg /kg without Epi 7 mg /kg with Epi 1:200K	Term neonates and infants: 1 mg/kg/hr
Bupivacaine or Ropivacaine	2–3 mg/kg	Term neonates: ≤0.2 mg/kg/hr 1–3 months: 0.25 mg/kg/hr Infants 3–6 months: 0.4 mg/kg/hr

Adapted from Sethna N, Suresh S. Central and peripheral regional analgesia and anaesthesia. In: Anand KJ et al. eds. *Pain in Neonates and Infants*, 3rd ed. Elsevier, 2007, p. 164.

Local Anesthetics

Local anesthetics are generally safe to use in pediatric populations, although excessive plasma concentrations can produce seizures and cardiac depression (1) [Table 10.2]. The commonly used local anesthetic agents are 2-chloroprocaine, lidocaine, bupivacaine, ropivacaine, mepivacaine, and tetracaine. The recent shortages in tetracaine and 2-chloroprocaine have limited their use recently. Due to low market demand, these agents are no longer being manufactured and are no longer available in the United States. The amino-amides have a narrower therapeutic index for neonates than for children or adults because of decreased metabolic clearance, with resultant drug accumulation during infusions, decreased plasma concentration of alpha-1-glycoprotein, and subsequently higher concentrations of unbound local anesthetic. Furthermore, it is difficult to recognize warning signs of impending toxic effects in preverbal neonates and infants (1).

Nonpharmacologic Management

Children are very responsive to pain-reducing strategies that involve their imagination and sense of play (21). Therefore, the involvement of child life specialists who are trained in a myriad of nonpharmacologic techniques is essential in the preparation of children preoperatively as well as in their pain management postoperatively.

Perioperative Pain Management in Elderly Populations

People are living longer, and this is reflected by the fact that the average age of the world's population is increasing rapidly, especially in the population greater than 80 years (22). Elderly patients undergo surgery four times more often than younger age groups, and thus healthcare practitioners should be well equipped to manage pain in these populations throughout the perioperative period (23). Conclusions from numerous studies have shown that older patients with pain do not receive effective pain management, whether the pain is acute or chronic (24). Elderly patients with dementia, those who are frail, or both, are more likely to have their pain undertreated, which can result in adverse outcomes such as poor sleep, impaired cognition, increased disability, depression, and reduced quality of life (25). Management of postoperative pain in older patients can be complicated by disease-related changes in physiology and disease–drug and drug–drug interactions. The evidence base for pain management in the elderly population remains limited because older patients, particularly those with significant medical comorbidities or cognitive impairment, are generally excluded from studies (24).

Assessment of Pain in Elderly Patients

Similar to children, assessment of perioperative pain in the elderly can be challenging due to barriers in reporting of pain, cognitive impairment, and difficulties in measurement. The reporting of pain in the elderly can vary with anxiety; depression; cognitive, visual, or hearing impairment; and social or family isolation associated with aging. Postoperative delirium occurs in 10% to 60% of patients, with a higher incidence in older patients (25). Cognitively intact older patients can reliably report their pain intensity with numeric rating scales, verbal descriptor scales, and also the Faces Pain Scale. In mild to moderately demented elderly patients the verbal descriptor scale is a better measure of pain. In patients with more advanced dementia or with significant postoperative delirium, observational measures of pain-related behaviors should be initiated if the previously mentioned methods have failed (24).

Analgesic Pharmacodynamic and Pharmacokinetic Considerations in the Elderly

Aging brings about physiologic, pharmacodynamic, and pharmacokinetic changes that should be taken into consideration when managing perioperative pain in the elderly (Table 10.3). The effects of aging on the central and peripheral nervous systems lead to a net loss of neurons in the cerebral cortex and the spinal cord, resulting in reduced neuronal conduction and increased sensitivity to local anesthetics (26). Elderly patients have increased fat mass and decreased muscle mass and body water, and this affects drug pharmacokinetics (27, 28). Hydrophilic drugs have a smaller volume of distribution as a consequence of these changes, resulting in higher plasma concentrations at equivalent doses and leading to a higher frequency of adverse effects. Lipophilic drugs, such as fentanyl and lidocaine, will have an increased volume of distribution that may prolong the duration of effect (29, 30). Elderly patients also have reduced liver size and blood flow, which can affect phase I catalysis more than phase II conjugation (29) and can decrease both total drug clearance and free drug clearance (29, 31). A decrease in the serum albumin concentration can be seen in elderly patients. This can lead to a reduction in the degree of plasma protein binding of drugs and an increase in the free drug in the plasma (24), especially with NSAIDs, many local anesthetics, and opioids, which are highly protein-bound (3). The most significant organ changes occur in the aging kidneys (29): the elderly present with decreased glomerular filtration rate, tubular excretion, tubular reabsorption, renal metabolism, and clearance of medications and metabolites (3).

Non-Opioids

The maximum recommended dose of acetaminophen of 4 g/day is generally well tolerated by elderly patients. Currently, there is no clear evidence that aging affects the clearance of acetaminophen, although commonly the dose is decreased prophylactically in clinical practice (3, 24).

Table 10.3 Pharmacodynamic and Pharmacokinetic Considerations in the Elderly

System	Functional Change	Clinical Consequence
Cardiac	↓ Cardiac output	↓ Sympathetic response following epidural/spinal anesthesia, ↓ cardiac output of 0–20% can lead to higher peak arterial concentrations of opioids after IV administration (24)
Hepatic	↓ Phase I metabolism ↓ Blood flow, ↓ Liver mass	↓ Hepatic metabolism of drugs with a high extraction ration (e.g., opioids and lidocaine) (24)
Renal	↓ Glomerular filtration rate, ↓ clearance	↑ Plasma concentrations of renally cleared drugs (e.g., NSAIDs) and metabolites (e.g., morphine) (23)
Central/peripheral nervous system	Net loss of neurons	↓ Conduction velocity through peripheral nervous system, ↑ Sensitivity to local anesthetics with neuraxial and peripheral nerve blocks
Muscular	↓ Muscle mass, ↑ body fat	↑ Volume of distribution and duration of lipophilic drugs
Pulmonary	↓ Respiratory center sensitivity	↑ Incidence of ventilatory depression (e.g., opioids, regional techniques)

NSAIDs are culpable for a large proportion of elderly patients who are hospitalized secondary to adverse reactions (23). These patients often have cardiovascular disease and an age-related decline in renal function and take multiple medications that can potentially interact with NSAIDs (30). Older patients are at high risk for renal complications following nonselective NSAID administration. The incidence of renal failure increases in the presence of preexisting renal impairment, low serum albumin levels, hypovolemia, hypotension, and concomitant medications, including NSAIDs and diuretics or angiotensin-converting enzyme inhibitors and other nephrotoxic agents. In the elderly, the dose of nonselective NSAIDs should be reduced by 25% to 50% and the dosing intervals should be increased. Nonselective NSAIDs are contraindicated in the postoperative period if the estimated creatinine clearance is less than 50 mL/min (23, 24).

Elderly patients are at greater risk of gastrointestinal (GI) adverse effects, including ulcers, bleeding, and perforation. The risk of GI bleeding from the use of nonselective NSAIDs is approximately twice as high in patients older than 65. The mortality from peptic ulcers is also much greater in the elderly (23, 24, 28).

Notable risk factors associated with GI injury are age greater than 70 years and the concurrent use of aspirin, even at smaller cardioprotective doses (24). NSAIDs can have pharmacokinetic and pharmacodynamic interactions with other drugs. Warfarin administered concurrently with a COX-2 inhibitor or a nonselective NSAID can increase the risk of GI bleeding 1.7-fold and 3.6-fold, respectively, compared with warfarin alone (28). Selective serotonin reuptake inhibitors can affect platelet function when used in combination with NSAIDs and have been associated with a 6-fold increase in the risk of GI bleeding when compared with untreated patients (28). Other medications that can increase the risk of GI injury and bleeding in the elderly include corticosteroids, low-molecular-weight heparin, and herbal products, particularly ginkgo biloba (24, 28).

Epidemiologically, patients taking COX-2 selective NSAIDs have an increased rate of GI complications compared with patients not taking NSAIDs. NSAIDs, particularly COX-2 inhibitors, are also associated with an increased risk of myocardial infarction (28).

Opioids

Opioids can also be used to treat pain in the elderly (23) (Table 10.4). A reduced dose of opioids is generally recommended in the elderly because of age-related changes in pharmacokinetics and pharmacodynamics. A 50% reduction in clearance, a reduction in protein binding, and increased brain sensitivity to the effects of opioids can be seen in older patients (31). Patient age rather than patient weight can be a better clinical predictor of postoperative opioid requirement, as there is an inverse relationship between average opioid dose and age. Despite this, there remains significant interindividual variation in opioid requirements in older patients; therefore, opioids must be titrated for each patient to achieve adequate analgesia (3, 23, 29).

Morphine is a commonly used opioid in the perioperative period. Its volume of distribution is decreased by 50% in older patients. The elimination of morphine's active metabolites is decreased subsequent to the decreased glomerular filtration commonly exhibited in the elderly (3, 23, 24, 29, 32). An increase in opioid metabolites and associated increased adverse effects can be seen with all of the commonly used opioids except fentanyl and buprenorphine (23, 24, 30). In particular, meperidine hydrochloride should be avoided in patients with renal impairment because its metabolite can result in significant neurotoxicity (33). Liver conjugation, a main form of opioid metabolism, is relatively well preserved in elderly patients despite age-related decreases in hepatic function (23).

Studies also show that the elderly have a great likelihood of respiratory depression than younger patients (31); therefore, proper monitoring and safeguards should be in place. Additionally, cognitive impairment, delirium, and hallucinations may occur with opioids, most commonly with meperidine but also with morphine and hydromorphone (31). Other side effects of opioids seen in younger patients, such as nausea, vomiting, and pruritus, are less common in the elderly (23).

IV-PCA in Elderly Populations

PCA can be a safe and effective method of providing perioperative analgesia for cognitively intact elderly patients (23). Standard opioid considerations and precautions should be taken into account when treating these patients.

Neuraxial Analgesia

Patient-controlled epidural analgesia in elderly patients has been shown to provide greater pain relief and satisfaction than IV-PCA (34). However, practitioners must be aware that older patients are more sensitive to the effects of local anesthetics administered through an epidural. The concentration of equal volumes of local anesthetics to achieve an effective motor blockade decreases with patient age (23, 24). According to a study by Simon and colleagues (35),

Table 10.4 Pharmacokinetics of Analgesics in the Elderly

Drug	Type	Volume of Distrubution	Clearance	Duration of Effect	Other Comments
Fentanyl (sufentanil, alfentanil)	Lipophilic Protein-bound	←	→	←	
Morphine	Hydrophilic Protein-bound	→	→	←	↑ Frequency of adverse effects
Local anesthetics	Amphipathic (lipophilic and hydrophilic components)	←	→	←	↓ Peak plasma levels due to decreased systemic absorption
Ketamine	NMDA-R antagonist Lipophilic Low protein-binding	←	→	↔ / ↑	CYP450 clearance; NMDA-R antagonists improve function in patients with Alzheimer's disease (24)
NSAIDs	Lipophilic Protein-bound	←	→	↔	

older patients experience bradycardia and hypotension more frequently than younger patients after administration of epidural ropivacaine. The elderly have decreased hepatic blood flow and a reduced mean clearance of local anesthetics, increasing their susceptibility to the toxic effects of local anesthetics if plasma concentrations reach significantly high levels during continuous epidural administration (34). Elderly patients are at high risk of developing postoperative cognitive decline and delirium. In a systematic review comparing the effects of common postoperative pain-management techniques on postoperative cognitive status, it was concluded that IV versus epidural techniques do not influence cognitive function differently (36).

Intrathecal analgesia is often used in the elderly, especially those undergoing orthopaedic, genitourologic, abdominal, and gynecologic procedures. Elderly patients have decreased physiologic reserve and a higher incidence of systemic disease, which makes them particularly vulnerable and at higher risk of experiencing bradycardia and hypotension following spinal neural blockade (37). The effects of profound hypotension, especially after high dermatome blockade that can be seen following spinal analgesia, can have severely detrimental effects in elderly patients with limited cardiac reserve (37). Neuraxial analgesia with epidural and intrathecal techniques can be challenging in this population because patient positioning and needle entry may be more difficult than in younger patients (38). Intrathecal analgesia adjuvants, such as clonidine and opioids, have been used in the elderly to increase the intensity and duration of neural blockade (38). Side effects are similar to epidural analgesia and must be considered when initiating intrathecal analgesia. Because elderly patients may be anticoagulated for various conditions, standard guidelines regarding anticoagulation and neuraxial analgesia must be followed (39).

Regional Techniques

Peripheral nerve blocks are an increasingly common technique for perioperative pain control for a wide variety of procedures. Performing these blocks in the elderly can be technically challenging due to arthritic changes that may interfere with positioning. Conversely, bony landmarks in the elderly are generally easily identifiable (36). Peripheral nerve blocks in the elderly have a higher risk of producing neurologic complications, including persistent numbness and nerve palsies (40). In a systemic review, regional anesthesia did not reduce the incidence of postoperative delirium and cognitive impairment compared with general anesthesia (41). However, peripheral nerve blocks for postoperative pain in the elderly can provide excellent analgesia and help avert some of the adverse effects associated with opioids (24).

Conclusion

Perioperative pain management in the elderly and children can be challenging. Fortunately, there are a variety of analgesic modalities to choose from to provide a multimodal approach to treating pain safely in these populations. This chapter has given an overview of currently accepted modalities of perioperative pain management in these populations, although much remains to be discovered and studied in the treatment of pain in these populations.

References

1. Coldrey J, Upton R, Macintyre P. Advances in analgesia in the older patient. *Best Pract Res Clin Anaesthesiol* 2011;25:367–378.

2. Berde C, Sethna NF. Analgesics for the treatment of pain in children. *N Engl J Med* 2002;347(14):1094–1103.

3. McLachlan AJ, Bath S, Naganathan V, Hilmer SN, Le Couteur DG, Gibson SJ, Blyth FM. Clinical pharmacology of analgesic medications of frailty and cognitive impairment. *Br J Clin Pharmacol* 2010;71(3):351–364.

4. Schechter NL, Allen DA, Hanson K. Status of pediatric pain control: A comparison of hospital analgesic usage in children and adults. *Pediatrics* 1986;77:11–15.

5. Schechter NL, Berde CB, Yaster M. Pain in infants, children and adolescents: An overview. In: Schechter NL, Berde CB, Yaster M, eds. *Pain in Infants, Children and Adolescents*, 2nd ed. Philadelphia: Lippincott Williams & Wilkins, 2003:3.

6. Fitzgerald M, Beggs S. The neurobiology of pain: developemental aspects. *Neuroscientist* 2001;7:246–257.

7. Klimach VJ, Cooke RW. Maturation of the neonatal somatosensory evoked response in preterm infants. *Dev Med Child Neurol* 1988;30:208–214.

8. Pattison D, Fitzgerald M. The neurobiology of infant pain; development of excitatory and inhibitory neurotransmission in the spinal dorsal horn. *Reg Anesth Pain Med* 2004;29(1):36–44.

9. Porter FL, Grunau RE, Anand KJ. Long-term effects of pain in infants. *J Dev Behav Pediatr* 1999;20:253–261.

10. Franck LS, Greenberg CS, Stevens B. Pain assessment in infants and children. *Pediatr Clin North Am* 2000;47(3):487–512.

11. Bieri D, Reeve RA, Champion GD, et al. The Faces Pain Scale for the self assessment of the severity of pain experienced by children: development, initial validation, and preliminary investigation for ration scale properties. *Pain* 1990;41(2):139–150.

12. McClain BC, Lee BH. Applied pharmacology in pediatric pain management. *Curr Rev Pain* 1997;1:296–309.

13. Jones V. Acetaminophen injection: A review of clinical information. *J Pain Palliative Care Pharmacotherapy*. 2011;25:340–349.

14. Jahr J, Lee V. Intravenous acetaminophen. *Anesthesiol Clin* 2010;28:619–645.

15. Verghese ST, Hannallah RS. Acute pain management in children. *J Pain Res* 2010;3:105–123.

16. Møiniche S, Rømsing J, Dahl J, Trame`r M. Nonsteroidal antiinflammatory drugs and the risk of operative site bleeding after tonsillectomy: a quantitative systematic review. *Anesth Analg* 2003;96:68–77.

17. Martin R, DiFiore J, Jana L, Davis R, Miller M, Coles S, Dick T. Persistence of biphasic ventilatory response to hypoxia in preterm infants. *J Pediatr* 1998;132(6):960–964.

18. Ameritage EN. Local anaesthetic techniques for prevention of postoperative pain. *Br J Anesth* 1986;58:790–800.

19. Moriarty A. Pediatric epidural analgesia (PEA). *Pediatr Anesth*. 2012;22:51–55.

20. Suresh S, Wheeler M. Practical pediatric regional anesthesia. *Anesthesiol Clin North Am* 2002;20(1):83–113.

21. Varadarajan JL, Weisman SJ. Pediatric pain. In: Abram SE. *Pain Medicine: The Requisites in Anesthesiology*. Philadelphia: Mosby Elsevier, 2006:114–131.

22. Coldrey J, Upton R, Macintyre P. Advances in analgesia in the older patient. *Best Pract Res Clin Anaesthesiol* 2011;25:367–378.

23. Auburn F. The elderly patient and postoperative pain treatment. *Best Pract Res Clin Anaesthesiol* 2007;21(1):109–127.

24. Catananti C, Gambassi G. Pain assessment in the elderly. *Surg Oncol* 2010;19:140–148.

25. Barber JB, Gibson S. Treatment of chronic non-malignant pain in the elderly: safety considerations. *Drug Safety* 2009;32(6):457–474.

26. White P, White L, Monk T, et al. Perioperative care for the older outpatient undergoing ambulatory surgery. *Anesth Analg* 2012;114(6):1190–1215.

27. Aymanns C, Keller F, Maus S, Hartmann B, Czock D. Review on pharmacokinetics and pharmacodynamics and the aging kidney. *Clin J Am Soc Nephrol* 2010;5:314–327.

28. Kaye A, Baluch A, Scott J. Pain management in the elderly population: a review. *Ochsner Journal* 2010;10:179–187.

29. McLachlan A, Pont L. Drug metabolism in older people—A key consideration in achieving optimal outcomes with medicines. *J Gerontol A Biol Sci Med Sci* 2012;67A(2):175–180.

30. Barkin R, Beckerman M, Blum S, Clark F, Koh E. Wu D. Should nonsteroidal anti-inflammatory drugs (NSAIDs) be prescribed to the older adult? *Drugs Aging* 2010;27(10):775–789.

31. Auburn F, Mazoit J, Riou B. Postoperative intravenous morphine titration. *Br J Anaesth* 2012;108(2):193–201.

32. Rivera R, Antognini J. Perioperative drug therapy in elderly patients. *Anesthesiology* 2009;110:1176–1181.

33. Smith H, Bruckenthal P. Implications of opioid analgesia for medically complicated patients. *Drugs Aging* 2010;27(5):417–433.

34. Mann C, Pouzeratte, Eledjam J. Postoperative patient-controlled analgesia in the elderly. *Drugs Aging* 2003;20(5):337–345.

35. Simon M, Veering T, Stienstra R, van Kleef J, Burm A. The effects of age on neural blockade and hemodynamic changes after epidural anesthesia with ropivacaine. *Anesth Analg* 2002;94:1325–1330.

36. Fong H, Sands L, Leung J. The role of postoperative analgesia in delirium and cognitive decline in elderly patients: a systematic review. *Anesth Analg* 2006;102:1255–1266.

37. Veering B. Hemodynamic effects of central neural blockade in elderly patients. *Can J Anesth* 2006;53(2):117–121.

38. Tsui BC, Wagner A, Finucane B. Regional anaesthesia in the elderly: a clinical guide. *Drugs Aging* 2004;21(14):895–910.

39. Horlocker TT, et al. Regional anesthesia in the patient receiving antithrombotic or thrombolytic therapy: American Society of Regional Anesthesia and Pain Medicine Evidence-Based Guidelines, 3rd ed. *Reg Anesth Pain Med* 2010;35:64–101.

40. Silverstein J, et al. *Geriatric Anesthesiology.* New York: Springer, 2008.

41. Mason S, Noel-Storr A, Ritchie CW. The impact of general and regional anesthesia on the incidence of post-operative cognitive dysfunction and post-operative delirium: a systematic review with meta-analysis. *J Alzheimers Dis* 2010;22(3):67–79.

Chapter 11

Obstetric Pain

Alison Weisheipl and Richard D. Urman

Pain Pathways During Labor and Delivery

Labor and delivery pain is caused by contraction of the myometrium, which in turn dilates the cervix and causes distention of the perineum.

The first stage of labor is the period from the onset of labor to complete cervical effacement and dilation. The pain during this first stage of labor is visceral, originating from uterine contractions and cervical dilatation. Specifically, during the latent phase of the first stage of labor (onset of labor to 3–4 cm of dilation), the pain pathways involve the T11 to T12 dermatomes (1). During the active phase of the first stage of labor (3–4 cm of dilation to complete cervical dilation), the pain pathways eventually involve the T10-L1 dermatomes (1). Nulliparous women, women with dysmenorrhea, and women with fetopelvic disproportion tend to have higher perception of pain during the first stage of labor (2, 3).

The second stage of labor is the period from full cervical dilation to delivery of the neonate (1). Pain during the second stage of labor is largely from distention of pelvic and perineal structures (3). These somatic pain impulses travel via S2–4 via the pudendal nerve (3).

Methods of Analgesia for Labor and Delivery

Nonpharmacologic Techniques

Nonpharmacologic methods of pain relief during labor include alternative and psychological means such as massage, hydrotherapy, breathing techniques, hypnosis, acupuncture, and biofeedback (4). While there are very few maternal and fetal side effects associated with the nonpharmacologic techniques, they require prenatal education and training. Nonpharmacologic techniques can be used alone or as adjuncts to parenteral medications or neuraxial techniques.

Parenteral Medications

Opioids are the most commonly used parenteral medication to treat labor pain (3). A variety of opioid medications and doses are listed in Table 11.1. Use of systemic medications such as parenteral opioids is limited because they can readily cross the placenta and thus affect the fetus. Maternal respiratory depression and sedation, loss of maternal protective airway reflexes, delayed maternal

Table 11.1 Opioid Medications and Doses

Drug	Class	Common Dose	Onset	Duration	Comments
Morphine	Opioid agonist	5–10 mg IM 2–5 mg IV	20–40 min IM 3–5 min IV	3–4 hr	Neonatal respiratory depression
Hydromorphone	Opioid agonist	0.4–0.6 mg IV			Neonatal respiratory depression
Fentanyl	Opioid agonist	100 µg IM 25–50 µg IV	10 min IM 2–3 min IV	30–60 min	Neonatal respiratory depression, short duration of action
Remifentanil	Opioid agonist	0.05 µg/kg/min IV	1 min	6 min	Neonatal respiratory depression, very short duration of action
Meperidine	Opioid agonist	50–100 mg IM 25–50 mg IV	40–45 min IM 5–10 min IV	2–3 hr	Active metabolite with long half-life, neonatal depression
Nalbuphine	Opioid agonist–antagonist	10 mg IV/IM	15 min IM 2–3 min IV	3–6 hr	Ceiling analgesic effect
Midazolam	Benzodiazepine	1–2 mg IV	<1 min	15–20 min	Anterograde amnestic effect
Ketamine	NMDA antagonist	0.25 mg/kg IV	<1 min	3–5 min	Undesirable hypertension, amnesia, hallucinations

Data from references 2, 3, 5, 6

gastric emptying, and increased risk of neonatal depression limit the use of opioids for labor pain (3). Side effects tend to be dose-dependent rather than drug-dependent. While opioids can be administered in safe doses to provide some analgesia for the mother, these safe doses cannot reach the level of analgesia that regional techniques can achieve. Therefore, opioids are much more useful in labor as adjuncts to regional anesthetic techniques.

Although opioids are the most common systemic medication used for relief of labor pain, anxiolytics and NMDA antagonists are occasionally used. Midazolam and diazepam are benzodiazepines that rapidly cross the placenta to affect the fetus. The use of benzodiazepines during the first trimester may be associated with cleft lip malformations but there is inconclusive evidence about this adverse effect in the full-term fetus (5). Because of their potential to cause prolonged neonatal depression as well as their potent amnestic properties, the use of benzodiazepines in labor is limited (3).

Ketamine is an NMDA receptor antagonist that can produce dissociative analgesia with minimal respiratory depression. It has a quick onset and short duration (see Table 11.1). However, ketamine has undesirable side effects such as hypertension and possible amnesia and can cause profound hallucinations and dreams (5). Ketamine may also increase uterine tone in high doses (>2mg/kg) (5). Because of its amnestic properties and potential for hallucinations, ketamine can have a negative impact on the labor experience for the mother. Similar to opioids, ketamine is much more useful in labor as an adjunct to regional techniques.

Regional Analgesia

Epidural

Epidural analgesia is the administration of local anesthetics and/or opioid analgesics to the epidural space via an epidural catheter. A test dose of local anesthetic is given after placement of the epidural to identify accidental intrathecal injection. Addition of epinephrine to the local anesthetic test dose can help to identify intravascular injection but is controversial as it may decrease uteroplacental perfusion (7). Epidurals can provide segmental bands of analgesia for the first stage of labor, and the block can be extended to provide analgesia for the second stage of labor (3). With epidural techniques, profound analgesia is achieved with minimal respiratory or cognitive depressant effects on the mother and fetus, and overall maternal catecholamine concentrations are reduced (3).

Labor epidural analgesia utilizes local anesthetics either alone or with opioids (3, 8). It has been suggested that epidural opioids and local anesthetic solutions work synergistically by acting on different sites of action (opioid receptors and neuronal axons, respectively) (9). When combined, lower concentrations of both local anesthetics and opioids can be used to reduce the incidence of adverse side effects (3, 10). If the opioid is omitted, higher concentrations of the local anesthetic are required, which can lead to motor block and impair the parturient's ability to push effectively (3). Similarly, if the local anesthetic is omitted, the dose of fentanyl needed to attain moderate analgesia is associated with side effects such as maternal sedation or neonatal depression (3). Table 11.2 discusses initiation and maintenance dosing of epidurals.

Spinal

Spinal analgesia is the administration of local anesthetics directly into the cerebrospinal fluid. Spinal analgesia can be given just prior to vaginal delivery to achieve a saddle block for vaginal delivery or it can be administered before cesarean section when a T4 sensory level is desired (3, 9). A single dose of local anesthetic with or without opioid is administered to the intrathecal space via a spinal needle. A 25- to 26-gauge pencil-point spinal needle is typically selected to decrease the risk of postdural puncture headache (3, 9). The duration of analgesia depends on the type of local anesthetic and opioid used and can be extended with the addition of vasoconstrictors such as epinephrine to the local

Table 11.2 Initiation and Maintenance Dosing of Epidurals

Solution	Local Anesthetic Concentration (mg/mL)	Opioid Concentration (µg/mL)	Volume (mL)
Epidural Initiation			
Bupivacaine	0.625–2.5	–	10–15
Bupivacaine + fentanyl	0.625–2.5	1–5	10–15
Bupivacaine + sufentantil	0.625–2.5	0.2–2	10–15
Epidural Maintenance			
Bupivacaine + fentanyl	0.625–1.25	2–4	
Bupivacaine + sufentanil	0.625–1.25	0.2–0.33	
Ropivacaine + fentanyl	0.8–1.0	2–4	
Ropivacaine	2.0		

Data from references 6, 9.

Table 11.3 Dosing of Spinal Analgesia for Cesarean Section

Drug	Dose	Notes
Fentanyl	10–25 µg	
Sufentanil	2.5–10 µg	
Morphine	0.20–0.30 mg	Requires special monitoring for delayed postoperative respiratory depression
Bupivacaine, hyperbaric	10–15 mg	

Data from references 6, 9.

anesthetic/opioid solution (3). Table 11.3 discusses dosing of spinal analgesia for cesarean section.

Combined Spinal-Epidural

Combined spinal-epidural (CSE) analgesia is the administration of local anesthetics into the intrathecal and epidural space. With vaginal deliveries, a CSE can benefit patients with severe pain in early or late labor (3, 6). For cesarean section, it combines the rapid and intense blockade achieved with spinal analgesia with the titration achieved with an epidural catheter (6). The epidural needle is used to locate the epidural space in loss-of-resistance fashion. Once the epidural space is located, a long spinal needle is passed through the epidural needle until the dura is punctured. Local anesthetic and/or opioids are administered in the intrathecal space, the spinal needle is removed, and an epidural catheter is then passed in the epidural space. The epidural infusion is started without a bolus dose. The patient has immediate analgesic effect from the administration of local anesthetic into the intrathecal space. However, with a CSE one cannot verify whether the epidural is functioning until the spinal has worn off.

Care should be taken when dosing epidural drugs because the epidural catheter may inadvertently penetrate the dura (6).

Contraindications to Neuraxial Analgesia

Patient refusal is the only absolute contraindication to neuraxial analgesia. Conditions such as severe hypovolemia, sepsis, infection at the site of needle insertion, coagulopathy, elevated intracranial pressures, and allergy to local anesthetics increase the risk of neuraxial analgesia. When these conditions arise, the risks and benefits must be weighed carefully (2).

Complications of Neuraxial Analgesia

Hypotension

The most common complication of neuraxial techniques for labor pain is hypotension (6), occurring as a result of sympathetic nervous system blockade. Maternal blood pressure and heart rate should be monitored at 5-minute intervals for at least 15 to 20 minutes after the blockade (9). Hypotension can be effectively treated with intravenous fluid administration and/or administration of a vasopressor. Leftward displacement of the uterus should be applied to avoid aortocaval compression (3).

Unintentional Intravascular Injection

Unintentional intravascular injection of local anesthetic can present as central nervous system excitation (seizures) or cardiac collapse (6). Early recognition of intravascular local anesthetic injection can be detected by the use of small incremental doses. If seizure develops, maintaining a patent airway and adequate oxygenation are necessary to prevent hypoxemia, hypercarbia, and acidosis (3). Barbiturates and benzodiazepines may also be useful to treat seizures. Cardiac resuscitation can be difficult after bupivacaine-induced cardiotoxicity because of the slower dissociation from sodium channels compared to lidocaine (3). ACLS should be initiated, but there are no specific recommendations for treating bupivacaine-induced cardiotoxicity. Lipid emulsion therapy has been documented in case studies as a method of treatment for refractory cardiac arrest (11).

Unintentional Intrathecal Injection

Accidental subarachnoid injection of local anesthetic can result in a high or total spinal. Hypotension, complete sensory and motor blockade, apnea, loss of protective airway reflexes, and unconsciousness can result (6). Treatment is supportive and includes endotracheal intubation. Vasopressor administration should be considered if supportive measures are not effective (2).

Postdural Puncture Headache

Postdural puncture headache is a result of inadvertent puncture of the subarachnoid space during the placement of an epidural catheter. Unintentional dural puncture occurs in about 3% of epidural placements in laboring women, with 70% of women with a dural puncture experiencing a severe headache (10). Postdural puncture headache can also occur in the setting of spinal anesthesia; the use of a 25g Whitacre needle for spinal anesthesia results in a similar rate of postdural puncture headache as compared to epidural anesthesia (3). Treatment includes caffeine, or in the event of severe refractory headache an epidural blood patch can be placed (6). Fifteen to 20 mL of autologous blood is sterilely placed into the epidural space near the level of the dural puncture. Headache relief is achieved in more than 75% of women (10).

Altered Progression of Labor

The progress of labor is variable and unpredictable. Parity, fetus presentation, and maternal pain all influence labor progression (3). Early analgesia via regional or parenteral routes could be a sign of women who would otherwise experience prolonged or dysfunctional labor (12). After labor has become active, neuraxial techniques do not prolong the first stage of labor. However, neuraxial techniques can remove the woman's ability to bear down during the second stage of labor and thus may prolong the second stage of labor (13). The decision to continue to observe versus operative delivery in the second stage is dependent on the fetal and maternal well-being (3).

References

1. Urman RD, Vadivelu N, eds. *Pocket Pain Medicine*. Philadelphia: Lippincott Williams & Wilkins. 2011.

2. Barash PG, Cullen BF, Stoelting RK, eds. *Clinical Anesthesia*, 6th ed. Philadelphia: Lippincott Williams & Wilkins. 2006.

3. Chestnut DH, Polley LS, Tsen LC, Wong CA, eds. *Chestnut's Obstetric Anesthesia: Principles and Practice*, 4th ed. Philadelphia: Mosby Elsevier, 2009.

4. Eappen S, Robbins D. Nonpharmacological means of pain relief for labor and delivery: A review. *Int Anesthesiol Clin* 2002;40(4):103–114.

5. Miller RD, ed. *Miller's Anesthesia*, 7th ed. Philadelphia: Elsevier Churchill Livingstone, 2009.

6. Hughes SC, Levinson G, Rosen MA, eds. *Shnider and Levinson's Anesthesia for Obstetrics*, 4th ed. Philadelphia: Lippincott Williams & Wilkins, 2002.

7. Mulroy M, Glosten B. The epinephrine test dose in obstetrics: Note the limitations. *Anesth Analg* 1998;86(5):923–925.

8. Camann W. Pain relief during labor. *N Engl J Med* 2005;352(7):718–720.

9. Morgan GE, Mikhail MS, Murray MJ. *Clinical Anesthesiology*, 4rd ed. New York: McGraw Hill, 2006.

10. Eltzschig HK, Lieberman ES, Camann WR. Regional anesthesia and analgesia for labor and delivery. *N Engl J Med* 2003;348(4):319–332.

11. Rosenblatt MA, Able M, Fischer GW, et al. Successful use of a 20% lipid emulsion to resuscitate a patient after a presumed bupivacaine-related cardiac arrest. *Anesthesiology* 2006;105(1):217–218.

12. Wong CA, Scavone BM, Peaceman AM, et al. The risk of cesarean delivery with neuraxial analgesia given early versus late in labor. *N Engl J Med* 2005;352 (7):655–665

13. Segal S. Epidural analgesia and the progress and outcome of labor and delivery. *Int Anesthesiol Clin* 2002;40(4):13–26

Chapter 12

Outcomes and Future Directions

Nathaniel Pleasant, Amitabh Gulati, and Roniel Weinberg

Introduction

Image guidance has expanded our regional anesthesia techniques. Adjuvant medications to standard acute pain treatment options have improved pain scores and decreased side effects. Also, new formulations of local anesthetics may improve our regional anesthesia outcomes and duration of action.

Image Guidance in Regional Anesthesia

In the past 15 years we have seen a tremendous increase in the role of ultrasound guidance in regional anesthesia as the preferred method for nerve localization. The majority of outcome data expounding the benefits of ultrasound in regional anesthesia has been from small-scale studies with limited patient populations (1). Meta-analysis comparing ultrasound-guided and nerve stimulation techniques have shown that ultrasound-guided blocks take less time to perform and demonstrate higher success rates, faster onset, and longer duration times (2). Unfortunately, the low incidence of complications (as low as 0.002%) makes it difficult to effectively estimate neural injury associated with ultrasound-guided nerve blocks (1, 3).

Ultrasound guidance allows the direct visualization of the targeted nerve, the needle trajectory, the spread of local anesthetic, and the surrounding anatomic structures. It allows practitioners to determine the minimum effective local anesthetic dose for various nerve blocks (4, 5). While theoretically a lower local anesthetic dose seems safer, there is little evidence that reducing the amount of local anesthetic reduces the frequency of local anesthetic systemic toxicity (6).

Intraneural injection of local anesthetic has traditionally been avoided during regional anesthesia, but recent reports have challenged this notion (7–9). In an evaluation of 24 patients receiving intraneural popliteal sciatic nerve blocks with pressures less than 20 psi, Robards and colleagues demonstrated adequate surgical anesthesia in all 24 patients and no cases of associated neurologic dysfunction (9). While there are case studies of neurologic symptoms after incidental intraneural injection of local anesthetic, many reports in animal models have failed to demonstrate any detrimental effect of intraneural injection on nerve motor function (10, 11).

With the practice of ultrasound for nerve blocks becoming standard, guidelines and structured training requirements in education are paramount (12). Studies evaluating the learning curve of anesthesiology residents show that novice practitioners can rapidly develop proficient skills in the use of ultrasound for regional anesthesia (13, 14). Common mistakes include poor choice of needle-insertion site, failure to recognize erroneous distribution of injected local anesthetic, and failure to visualize the needle before movement.

Advances in Adjuvant Pharmacotherapy for Acute Pain

In the continuing effort to manage pain more effectively while minimizing the adverse effects of opioids, drugs such as intravenous (IV) acetaminophen, IV nonsteroidal anti-inflammatories (NSAIDs), and GABA analogs have been given preoperatively for pain control.

IV acetaminophen has been shown to improve pain relief and decrease opioid consumption by 20% compared with placebo in two meta-analyses (15, 16). Despite showing diminished opioid use, these studies have not demonstrated reduction of opioid-induced side effects such as postoperative nausea and vomiting (17–19). IV acetaminophen has a more predictable time to peak effect than the oral or rectal form but has not been associated with more effective pain control compared to the other routes of administration and may be more expensive (19).

IV ibuprofen was approved for use in the United States in 2009 and has been evaluated in several multicenter trials (20–22). In patients following either orthopaedic or abdominal surgeries, an IV dose of 800 mg ibuprofen demonstrated decreased morphine use during the first 24 hours (22% vs. placebo, p = .030) and reduced pain at rest (30.6% vs. placebo, p < .001) (20). The use of IV ibuprofen as a preemptive analgesic in patients undergoing orthopaedic surgery demonstrated a reduction in morphine requirements during the postoperative period (30.9% vs. placebo, p < .001), decreased pain at rest (31.8% vs. placebo, p < .001), and decreased pain with movement (25.8% vs. placebo, p < .001) (21). The use of IV ibuprofen has been shown to have an opioid-sparing effect of up to 50%, consequently reducing the incidence of opioid-associated sedation and related emetic episodes by as much as 30% (23). The combination of an NSAID and acetaminophen offers superior analgesia compared to either modality alone (24).

Anticonvulsants have traditionally been used in the treatment of chronic neuropathic pain, and now they are used in perioperative pain control. In a systematic review of 16 studies, a single preoperative dose of gabapentin 1,200 mg decreased pain scores at 6 and 24 hours following surgery and reduced cumulative opioid consumption and side effects during the first 24 hours postoperatively (25). In patients undergoing mastectomy, a single preoperative dose of 1,200 mg gabapentin decreased postoperative morphine use from a median of 29 mg to 15 mg (p < .001) and pain intensity associated with movement (26). However, postoperative administration of gabapentin in patients undergoing total abdominal hysterectomy found minimal reduction in pain during the acute postoperative period, but showed decreased chronic pain associated with the procedure (27).

In patients undergoing major spinal surgery, 300 mg pregabalin given preoperatively and 150 mg given twice daily for 48 hours postoperatively demonstrated reduced morphine consumption ($p < .05$) and a lower incidence of postoperative constipation and nausea/vomiting (28). A meta-analysis of 22 studies showed that pregabalin administered during the perioperative period results in lower analgesic drug consumption postoperatively (29). The study determined similar efficacy for doses of 225 to 300 mg/day and 600 to 750 mg/day, but no effect at doses of 150 mg/day. Another trial demonstrated no clinical benefit from perioperative administration of pregabalin (100 mg given preoperatively, 50 mg q12h for 3 days postoperatively) as part of a multimodal analgesic regimen following foot and ankle surgery (30).

Future Directions for Local Anesthetics

Local anesthetics, a staple of perioperative regional analgesic regimens, help increase postoperative analgesia while decreasing consumption of opioids. Recent research efforts have prolonged the effects of local anesthetics. Adjuvants, such as dexamethasone, to local anesthetics have also shown some synergy in neural blockade.

Recent clinical studies have shown prolongation of analgesia with the addition of dexamethasone to local anesthetics in peripheral nerve blocks. Patients who received interscalene brachial plexus blocks for shoulder arthroscopy showed prolongation of median sensory (1457 vs. 833 minutes) and motor (1374 vs. 827 minutes) blockade with the addition of 8 mg dexamethasone versus placebo to a mixture of bupivacaine 0.5% with epinephrine and clonidine (31). Similarly, 8 mg of dexamethasone added to 0.5% ropivacaine and bupivacaine prolonged the analgesic effect of each to about 22 hours (32). In addition, dexamethasone has been shown to prolong the median duration of analgesia (332 vs. 228 minutes) when combined with 30 cc of 1.5% mepivacaine in supraclavicular brachial plexus blockade (33). None of these studies showed neurotoxicity or side effects from the addition of dexamethasone (34).

Biotoxins, such as saxitoxin from dinoflagellates and tetrodotoxin from fugu puffer fish, are sodium channel-blocking agents that may be used similarly as local anesthetics (35). Their use has been limited by toxicity, neuronal blockade, and muscular weakness with resultant diaphragmatic paralysis, respiratory arrest, and death (36). However, studies with epinephrine or bupivacaine combined with tetrodotoxin produced prolonged sciatic blockade in rats while decreasing systemic toxicity and increasing the median lethal dose (36). Comparing neosaxitoxin (derivative of saxitoxin) to bupivacaine via port infiltration for laparoscopic cholecystectomy showed that neosaxitoxin led to significantly lower pain scores at 12 hours postoperatively, with no serious adverse effects and a lower risk of neurotoxicity and myotoxicity compared to amino-amide local anesthetics (37, 38). Other animal toxins, such as ralfinamide; ProTx-II (peptide from venom of the tarantula), which inhibits sodium channels on C nerve fibers; and ziconotide, which blocks N-type calcium channels at presynaptic primary afferent nerve terminals, have potential applications in regional anesthesia (39).

Encapsulation of local anesthetics with liposomes may increase their duration and decrease systemic toxicity (35). Water-soluble drug can be carried in the central compartment, lipid-soluble drug in the lipid bilayer (39). ExaprelTM (Pacira Pharmaceuticals Inc., NJ, USA) uses the Depofoam® drug-delivery system containing bupivacaine. The nonencapsulated bupivacaine has an immediate effect upon injection, while the encapsulated bupivacaine is released over time through reorganization of the lipid membranes (40).

The efficacy of wound infiltration with liposomal bupivacaine has been studied in patients undergoing breast augmentation, hemorrhoidectomy, hernia repair, knee arthroplasty, and bunionectomy (41–46). Liposomal bupivacaine provided reduction of pain, decreased opioid use, prolonged time to first opioid use, and improved patient satisfaction through 72 hours (43). A pooled analysis of efficacy data from phase 2 and phase 3 randomized double-blind trials showed liposomal bupivacaine at 72 hours to be associated with lower pain scores than the control arms in 16 of 19 treatment arms (41). An assessment of the cardiac safety profile of liposomal extended-release bupivacaine revealed no prolongation of the QTc interval or other cardiac safety issues at doses up to 750 mg (47).

DepoDur®, which utilizes the Depofoam® drug-delivery system with morphine, has been used safely for over a decade to provide epidural analgesia (44). An early, small, nonrandomized controlled study showed an almost 100% increased time to analgesia with liposomal 0.5% bupivacaine compared to plain 0.5% bupivacaine with 1:200,000 epinephrine (48).

Conclusion

Efforts are under way to improve our delivery of regional anesthesia and adjuvant medications to improve acute pain treatment outcomes. Imaging and pharmacotherapy options will improve our quality of care in the acute pain patient.

References

1. Marhofer P, Chan VW. Ultrasound-guided regional anesthesia: current concepts and future trends. *Anesth Analg* 2007;104(5):1265–1269.

2. Abrahams MS, Aziz MF, Fu RF, Horn J-L. Ultrasound guidance compared with electrical neurostimulation for peripheral nerve block: a systematic review and meta-analysis of randomized controlled trials. *Br J Anaesth* 2009;102(3):408–417.

3. Auroy Y, Benhamou D, Bargues L, et al. Major complications of regional anesthesia in France: the SOS Regional Anesthesia Hotline Service. *Anesthesiology* 2002;97:1274–1280.

4. Duggan E, El Beheiry H, Perlas A, Lupu M, Nuica A, Chan VW, Brull R. Minimum effective volume of local anesthetic for ultrasound-guided supraclavicular brachial plexus block. *Reg Anesth Pain Med* 2009;34(3):215–218.

5. Tran de QH, Dugani S, Correa JA, Dyachenko A, Alsenosy N, Finlayson RJ. Minimum effective volume of lidocaine for ultrasound-guided supraclavicular block. *Reg Anesth Pain Med* 2011;36(5):466–469.

6. Neal JM, Brull R, Chan VW, Grant SA, Horn J-L, Liu SS, et al. The ASRA evidence-based medicine assessment of ultrasound-guided regional anesthesia and pain medicine. *Reg Anesth Pain Med* 2010;35:S1–9.

7. Sala Blanch X, Lopez AM, Carazo J, Hadzic A, Carrera A, Pomes J, Valls-Sole J. Intraneural injection during nerve stimulator-guided sciatic nerve block at the popliteal fossa. *Br J Anaesth* 2009;102:855–861.

8. Bigeleisen PE. Nerve puncture and apparent intraneural injection during ultrasound-guided axillary block does not invariably result in neurologic injury. *Anesthesiology* 2006;105:779–783.

9. Robards C, Hadzic A, Somasundaram L, Iwata T, Gadsden J, Xu D, Sala-Blanch X. Intraneural injection with low-current stimulation during popliteal sciatic nerve block. *Anesth Analg* 2009;109(2):673–677.

10. Chan VW, Brull R, McCartney CJ, Xu D, Abbas S, Shannon P. An ultrasonic and histological study of intraneural injection and electrical stimulation in pigs. *Anesth Analg* 2007;104(5):1281–1284.

11. Lupu Cm, Kiehl TR, Chan VW, El-Beheiry H, Madden M, Brull R. Nerve expansion seen on ultrasound predicts histologic but no functional nerve injury after intraneural injection in pigs. *Reg Anesth Pain Med* 2010;35:132–139.

12. Marhofer P, Harrop-Griffiths W, Kettner SC, Kirchmair L. Fifteen years of ultrasound guidance in regional anesthesia: Part 1. *Br J Anaesth* 2010;104(5):538–546.

13. Sites BD, Gallagher JD, Cravero J, Lundberg J, Blike G. The learning curve associated with a simulated ultrasound-guided interventional task by inexperienced anesthesia residents. *Reg Anesth Pain Med* 2004;29(6):544–548.

14. Sites BD, Spence BC, Gallagher JD, Wiley CW, Bertrand ML, Blike GT. Characterizing novice behavior associated with learning ultrasound-guided peripheral regional anesthesia. *Reg Anesth Pain Med* 2007;32(2):107–115.

15. Remy C, Marret E, Bonnet F. Effects of acetaminophen on morphine side-effects and consumption after major surgery: a meta-analysis of randomized controlled trials. *Br J Anaesth* 2005;94:505–513.

16. Elia N, Lysakowski C, Tramer M. Does multimodal analgesia with acetaminophen, nonsteroidal antiinflammatory drugs, or selective cyclooxygenase-2 inhibitors and patient-controlled analgesia morphine offer advantages over morphine alone? *Anesthesiology* 2005;103:1296–1304.

17. Arici S, Gurbet A, Turker G, Yavascaoglu B, Sahin S. Preemptive analgesic effects of intravenous paracetamol in total abdominal hysterectomy. *Agri.* 2009;21:54–61.

18. Hong JY, Kim WO, Chung WY, Yun JS, Kil HK. Paracetamol reduces postoperative pain and rescue analgesic demand after robot-assisted endoscopic thyroidectomy by the transaxillary approach. *World J Surg* 2010;34:521–526.

19. Capici F, Ingelmo PM, Davidson A, Sacchi, CA, Milan B, Rota Sperti L, Lorini L, Fumagalli R. Randomized controlled trial of duration of analgesia following intravenous or rectal acetaminophen after adenotonsillectomy in children. *Br J Anaesth* 2008;100(2):251–255.

20. Southworth S, Peters J, Rock A, Pavliv L. A multicenter, randomized, double-blind, placebo-controlled trial of intravenous ibuprofen 400 and 800 mg every 6 hours in the management of postoperative pain. *Clin Ther* 2009;31(9):1922–1935.

21. Singla N, Rock A, Pavliv L. A multi-center, randomized, double-blind placebo-controlled trial of intravenous-ibuprofen (IV-ibuprofen) for treatment of pain in post-operative orthopedic adult patients. *Pain Med* 2010;11(8):1284–1293.

22. Kroll PB, Meadows L, Rock A, Pavliv L. A multicenter, randomized, double-blind, placebo-controlled trial of intravenous ibuprofen (IV-ibuprofen) in the

management of postoperative pain following abdominal hysterectomy. *Pain Practice* 2011;11(1):23–32.

23. Marret E, Kurdi O, Zufferey P, Bonnet F. Effects of nonsteroidal antiinflammatory drugs on patient-controlled analgesia morphine side effects: meta-analysis of randomized controlled trials. *Anesthesiology* 2005;102:1249–1260.

24. Ong CK, Seymour RA, Lirk P, Merry AF. Combining paracetamol (acetaminophen) with nonsteroidal antiinflammatory drugs: a qualitative systematic review of analgesic efficacy for acute postoperative pain. *Anesth Analg* 2010;110(4):1170–1179.

25. Ho KY, Gan TJ, Habib AS. Gabapentin and postoperative pain: A systematic review of randomized controlled trials. *Pain* 2006;126:91–101.

26. Dirks J, Fredensborg BB, Christensen D, Fomsgaard JS, Flyger H, Dahl JB. A randomized study of the effects of single-dose gabapentin versus placebo on postoperative pain and morphine consumption after mastectomy. *Anesthesiology* 2002;97:560–564.

27. Fassoulaki A, Stamatakis, E, Petropoulos G, Siafaka I, Hassiakos D, Sarantopoulos C. Gabapentin attenuates late but not acute pain after abdominal hysterectomy. *Eur J Anaesthesiol* 2006; 23(2):136–141.

28. Gianesello L, Pavoni V, Barboni E, Galeotti I, Nella A. Perioperative pregabalin for postoperative pain control and quality of life after major spinal surgery. *J Neurosurg Anesthesiol* 2012;24(2):121–126.

29. Engelman E, Cateloy F. Efficacy and safety of perioperative pregabalin for postoperative pain; a meta-analysis of randomized-control trials. *Acta Anaesthesiol Scand.* 2011;55:927–943.

30. YaDeau JT, Paroli L, Kahn RL, et al. Addition of pregabalin to multimodal analgesic therapy following ankle surgery: a randomized double-blind, placebo-controlled trial. *Reg Anesth Pain Med* 2012;37:302–307.

31. Vieira PA, Pulai I, Tsao GC, Manikantan P, Keller B, Connelly NR. Dexamethasone with bupivacaine increases duration of analgesia in ultrasound-guided interscalene brachial plexus blockade. *Eur J Anaesthesiol* 2010;27(3):285–288.

32. Cummings KC 3rd, Napierkowski DE, Parra-Sanchez I, Kurz A, Dalton JE, Brems JJ, Sessler DI. Effect of dexamethasone on the duration of interscalene nerve blocks with ropivacaine or bupivacaine. *Br J Anaesth* 2011;107(3):446–453. doi: 10.1093/bja/aer159.

33. Parrington SJ, O'Donnell D, Chan VW, et al. Dexamethasone added to mepivacaine prolongs the duration of analgesia after supraclavicular brachial plexus blockade. *Reg Anesth Pain Med* 2010;35(5):422–426.

34. De la Fuente N, Altermatt FR. Adding dexamethasone to peripheral nerve blocks can give better postoperative analgesia. *Br J Anaesth* 2012;108(1):161–162.

35. Weiniger CF, Golovanevski L, Domb AJ, Ickowicz D. Extended release formulations for local anaesthetic agents. *Anaesthesia* 2012 May 18. doi: 10.1111/j.1365–2044.2

36. Kohane DS, Yieh J, Lu NT, Langer R, Strichartz GR, Berde CB. A re-examination of tetrodotoxin for prolonged duration local anesthesia. *Anesthesiology* 1998;89(1):119–131.

37. Rodr´guez-Navarro AJ, Berde CB, Wiedmaier G, et al. Comparison of neosaxitoxin versus bupivacaine via port infiltration for postoperative analgesia following laparoscopic cholecystectomy: a randomized, double-blind trial. *Reg Anesth Pain Med* 2011;36(2):103–109.

38. Rodriguez-Navarro AJ, Lagos N, Lagos M, et al. Intrasphincteric neosaxitoxin injection: evidence of lower esophageal sphincter relaxation in achalasia. *Am J Gastroenterol* 2006;101(11):2667–2668.

39. Wiles MD, Nathanson MH. Local anaesthetics and adjuvants—future developments. *Anaesthesia* 2010;65(Suppl 1):22–37.

40. Exaprel® (bupivacaine liposome injectable suspension) Product Monograph (online).

41. Bergese SD, Ramamoorthy S, Patou G, Bramlett K, Gorfine SR, Candiotti KA. Efficacy profile of liposome bupivacaine, a novel formulation of bupivacaine for postsurgical analgesia. *J Pain Res* 2012;5:107–116.

42. Minkowitz HS, Onel E, Patronella CK, Smoot JD. A two-year observational study assessing the safety of DepoFoam bupivacaine after augmentation mammaplasty. *Aesthet Surg J* 2012;32(2):186–193.

43. Gorfine SR, Onel E, Patou G, Krivokapic ZV. Bupivacaine extended-release liposome injection for prolonged postsurgical analgesia in patients undergoing hemorrhoidectomy: a multicenter, randomized, double-blind, placebo-controlled trial. *Dis Colon Rectum* 2011;54(12):1552.

44. Haas E, Onel E, Miller H, Ragupathi M, White PF. A double-blind, randomized, active-controlled study for post-hemorrhoidectomy pain management with liposome bupivacaine, a novel local analgesic formulation. *Am Surg* 2012;78(5):574–581.

45. Bramlett K, Onel E, Viscusi ER, Jones K. randomized, double-blind, dose-ranging study comparing wound infiltration of DepoFoam bupivacaine, an extended-release liposomal bupivacaine, to bupivacaine HCl for postsurgical analgesia in total knee arthroplasty. *Knee* 2012, doi:10.1016/j.knee.2011.12.004

46. Golf M, Daniels SE, Onel E. A phase 3, randomized, placebo-controlled trial of DepoFoam® bupivacaine (extended-release bupivacaine local analgesic) in bunionectomy. *Adv Ther* 2011;28(9):776–788. doi: 10.1007/s12325-011-0052-y

47. Bergese SD, Onel E, Morren M, Morganroth J. Bupivacaine extended-release liposome injection exhibits a favorable cardiac safety profile. *Reg Anesth Pain Med* 2012;37(2):145–151.

48. Boogaerts JG, Lafont ND, Declercq AG, et al. Epidural administration of liposome-associated bupivacaine for the management of postsurgical pain: a first study. *J Clin Anesth* 1994;6(4):315–320.

Index

123